# PLAY AND PLAYFULNESS FOR PUBLIC HEALTH AND WELLBEING

The role of play in human and animal development is well established, and its educational and therapeutic value is widely supported in the literature. This innovative book extends the play debate by assembling and examining the many pieces of the play puzzle from the perspective of public health. It tackles the dual aspects of art and science which inform both play theory and public health policy, and advocates for a 'playful' pursuit of public health, through the integration of evidence from parallel scientific and creative endeavors.

Drawing on international research evidence, the book addresses some of the major public health concerns of the 21st century – obesity, inactivity, loneliness and mental health – advocating for creative solutions to social disparities in health and wellbeing. From attachment at the start of life to detachment at life's ending, in the home and in the workplace, and across virtual and physical environments, play is presented as vital to the creation of a new 'culture of health'.

This book represents a valuable resource for students, academics, practitioners and policy-makers across a range of fields of interest including play, health, the creative arts and digital and environmental design.

**Alison Tonkin** is Head of Higher Education at Stanmore College, United Kingdom. Alison has a research background in health promotion for pre-school children and has worked as both a diagnostic and a therapeutic radiographer.

**Julia Whitaker** has worked therapeutically with children and families in both public and private sectors for the past 30 years. Originally trained as a social worker and family therapist, Julia is also a registered Health Play Specialist with wide-ranging clinical and teaching experience in the field.

Cover image courtesy of Lizzy Mikietyn, Edinburgh.

# PLAY AND PLAYFULNESS FOR PUBLIC HEALTH AND WELLBEING

*Edited by Alison Tonkin and Julia Whitaker*

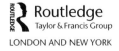

Routledge
Taylor & Francis Group

LONDON AND NEW YORK

First published 2019
by Routledge
2 Park Square, Milton Park, Abingdon, Oxon OX14 4RN

and by Routledge
52 Vanderbilt Avenue, New York, NY 10017

*Routledge is an imprint of the Taylor & Francis Group, an informa business*

*British Library Cataloguing in Publication Data*
A catalogue record for this book is available from the British Library

*Library of Congress Cataloging-in-Publication Data*
A catalog record has been requested for this book

ISBN: 978-1-138-54166-5 (hbk)
ISBN: 978-1-138-54168-9 (pbk)
ISBN: 978-1-351-01045-0 (ebk)

Typeset in Bembo
by Taylor & Francis Books

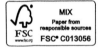

Printed and bound in Great Britain by
TJ International Ltd, Padstow, Cornwall

To Grinny and Pops:
with love and thanks for leaving a legacy of
play and playfulness
A.T.

To Freya and friends:
a playful future is yours for the making
J.W.

# CONTENTS

# ILLUSTRATIONS

Cover image courtesy of Lizzy Mikietyn, Edinburgh

## Figures

## Tables

# FOREWORD

When we think about play and playfulness we tend to think about children: the way in which they interact with each other and with adults to communicate, form relationships and simply enjoy the freedom of an activity that has no other purpose than having fun.

Public health might not be the first thing we associate with play, driven by science and much advice to change our lives, public health does not immediately bring to mind enjoyment. But the authors of this book have argued convincingly that we need to change the way we think about public health, to introduce playfulness into people's lives at all stages of the life course to strengthen the possibility for change.

Public health, the health of populations and communities, is at the heart of how countries, islands, cities, small communities and groups of people sustain their collective wellbeing, prevent disease and its spread and promote structural and political change to enable people to take up healthy lifestyles and engage in activities that will bring longer and happier lives. It has been recognised as a science since the 19th century when in England John Snow famously identified the link between contaminated water from a single pump in London and the spread of the great cholera epidemic. Other sanitary reformers such as Joseph Bazalgette contributed to major engineering projects in London that introduced a sewer system that is still in use, separating drinking water from the sewage that was disposed of and treated downriver. Vaccination against smallpox was discovered by Jenner and the technology of immunization developed for other infectious diseases during the 20th century so that in today's world we have the capability to immunize against a huge range of dangerous and infectious diseases. James Lind discovered the connection between scurvy and vitamin C deficiency, the Clean Air Acts removed the infamous smogs of London and more recently Julian Tudor Hart showed how careful data collection over time within a community could demonstrate patterns of ill health such as hypertension and help to make inferences between disease, lifestyle, demography and geography, the science of epidemiology. In 1920 the bacteriologist Charles-Edward Winslow founded Yale School of Public Health and captured his definition of public health:

> Public Health is the science and the art of preventing disease, prolonging life, and promoting physical health and efficiency through organized community efforts for the sanitation of the environment, the control of community infections, the education of the individual in principles of personal hygiene, the organization of medical and nursing service for the early diagnosis and preventive treatment of disease, and the development of the social machinery which will ensure to every individual in the community a standard of living adequate for the maintenance of health; organizing these benefits in such fashion as to enable every citizen to realize his birthright of health and longevity.

This definition has been drawn on by Tonkin and Whitaker, the editors of this book, to encapsulate all of the elements of public health, importantly because Winslow drew on the idea of *art* as well as *science*.

At one level the concept of public health appears to be so straightforward that it is difficult to argue against the proposition that 'prevention is better than cure'. If strategies and actions can be undertaken to prevent disease or injury and prolong life, and also save cost to countries and health systems, then why would policy focus more on sending ambulances to rescue people drowning downstream than building the necessary safety barriers upstream? It is perhaps this concept of upstream thinking that requires the kind of critical analysis that is part of the art of public health. After all, if the science and knowledge of preventive action were sufficient there would no longer be epidemics of preventable diseases such as measles or non-communicable causes of ill health such as obesity, many types of cancer, heart disease and mental health problems.

But these, among many other public health issues, persist across the globe and, as data from the World Health Organization and the World Bank demonstrate, there are huge inequalities between and within countries around the levels to which populations experience good public health.

One of the reasons for the persistence must be that the science turned during the 20th century away from structural and political change to individual behavior change. Despite global strategies such as Healthy Cities and Healthy Schools, the pressure was on individuals to take more responsibility for themselves and to change the way they eat, drink, exercise, relax, have sex, sleep, work, have children, use health services, every aspect of individual and family life has been the subject of scientific papers that aim to show how change will lead to health benefit. The world-wide obesity epidemic alone is testament to the fact that this approach just doesn't work. Public health and upstream thinking involves the art of understanding human factors, what makes people tick and how to deliver messages in ways that acknowledge challenges and limitations in everyday life as well as the positive benefits, and how people respond to scientific messages. Most recently, these ideas have been brought together through the Social Marketing approach, drawing on new technologies such as apps and online videos to 'nudge' and encourage people to do something different. Still, improvement in public health and inequality remains problematic.

In this book the editors have drawn on a different approach to the art of public health. Rather than demanding that people and communities change their behaviors and lifestyles against the odds of poverty, poor housing, unemployment, access to health care and availability of healthy environments they have chosen to focus on a concept that has no other purpose than pleasure and enjoyment: that of play.

Throughout the following chapters Tonkin and Whitaker uniquely build the case for drawing on play and playfulness as the central concepts for public health. What could be more refreshing than the idea that instead of being blamed for poor behavior, individuals, families and communities can explore ways to have fun, enjoy their lives through positive, playful interaction and activity and experience better health and wellbeing as a result? Drawing on a wide range of evidence from research, the authors build on the statement that 'Nothing lights up the brain like play' to show how the child and adolescent brain develops through play and the importance of play throughout life in promoting health and wellbeing.

Each chapter takes a different aspect of the life course - childhood, family life, disability, lived environment, social life and end of life to name some – and explores in detail how play and playfulness contribute to the salutogenic approach to public health. Salutogenesis is the production of good health, the antonym of pathogenesis the production of disease. The art of play and the art and creativity that comes through playfulness are counter-productive to pathogenesis and enable people to realize their strengths and assets through a new lens of upstream thinking.

I would recommend this book to everyone who is interested in positive and creative change and promoting healthy communities. There is scope for policy makers and commissioners to think about the structural and political environment that could enable more playful lives, for families, schools, communities to work and play together, for health services to consider a salutogenic, assets-based approach to supporting public health throughout the life course and for individuals to feel relieved from the pressure of difficult behavior interventions and to learn through play and creativity to improve wellbeing. Of course, this cannot be over-simplified, play and playfulness are serious and complex processes that have been critically investigated by researchers and which the authors draw on. There is no magic bullet for public health, but there are possibilities for everyone, everywhere to bring play and creativity into their lives.

Sally Kendall, MBE, PhD
Professor of Community Nursing and Public Health
Center for Health Services Studies
University of Kent at Canterbury, UK

# ACKNOWLEDGEMENTS

We would like to thank:

- All the contributors to this book who have added depth to the project through the generous sharing of their expertise.
- Professor Sally Kendall, for eloquently setting the scene with an informed commentary reflecting many years of public health expertise.
- Lizzy Mikietyn, for her vibrant cover illustration which so beautifully conveys the overriding message of this book.
- Grace McInnes, Commissioning Editor, Routledge, for giving us the opportunity to write this further exploration of play and playfulness linked to health and wellbeing.
- Carolina Antunes, Editorial Assistant, Health and Social Care, Routledge for trusting us to get on with the task in hand and completing the process with us.

Alison would like to thank:

- Julia, for sharing this journey with fun and friendship – the perfect combination.
- Nicola Conibear and the Senior Leadership Team at Stanmore College who enabled this project to be undertaken and completed under their care.
- Claire Weldon, for still listening and continuing to say 'yes'.
- My lovely family and friends who have, as always, been a constant source of love and patience, even when I am a #liability. A special mention for my baby bro Trev, because this will make you happy.

Julia would like to thank:

- Alison, for your energy and enthusiasm which have once again seen a plan brought to fruition.

- Morven Macrae, Eric Fleming and the Garvald Artists for allowing me to 'play, create, relate' with you.
- Grassroots organizations throughout the UK who continue to work tirelessly to keep play at the heart of childhood. A special shout-out to my friends @UpstartScotland.
- Freya, for all those morning cups of tea. Alex, for everything you do for us. I love you both.

Thanks to the following for giving permission to reproduce the figures that appear in this book: Professor Hugh Barton, Will Boex, Hannah Esnor, Annette Gossett, Jane McArthur, Dean Mendes, Lizzy Mikietyn, Earleatha Oppon, André Tomlin, AhHa Publications, Public Health England, the Government Office for Science and the Department of Health.

# CONTRIBUTORS

**Rachel Bayliss**, Intensive Care and Acute Medicine Fellow, Kings College Hospital.

**Jenni Etchells**, Specialist Children's Community Nurse and Clinical Practice Teacher (Freelance).

**Eric Fleming**, Social Therapy Craft Specialist, Garvald Edinburgh.

**Christina Freeman**, Professional Development Officer for the Society of Radiographers (retired).

**Alison Tonkin**, Head of Higher Education, Stanmore College.

**Claire Weldon**, Student Welfare Officer, Stanmore College.

**Julia Whitaker**, Health Play Specialist (Freelance); Registration Co-ordinator, Healthcare Play Specialist Education Trust.

**Lisa Whiting**, Professional Lead for Children's Nursing, University of Hertfordshire.

# INTRODUCTION

*Julia Whitaker and Alison Tonkin*

The role of play in human and animal development is well established (Brown 2008), and its educational and therapeutic value is widely supported in the literature (White-bread 2012). This book extends the play debate by assembling and examining the many pieces of the play puzzle from the perspective of public health. It is presented as a further contribution to the growing social movement to elevate the status of play in the lives of individuals, communities and of society as a whole, by addressing the diverse and extensive appreciation of the role of public health as we move through the 21st century.

In 2011, musician, author and social commentator Pat Kane famously pronounced: 'Play will be to the 21st century what work was to the industrial age – our dominant way of knowing, doing and creating value' (Kane 2012). In many ways, play is in the ascendant.

As the manuscript for this book approached completion, the American Association of Pediatrics published a report (Yogman et al. 2018) reinforcing the importance of play for child development and recommending the 'prescription' of play as a counterbalance to the increasingly didactic focus of early education, the over-scheduling of free time, and the insidious control of digital media. In the same week, the BBC published a feature on 'the rise of the adult toy fans' (Peachey 2018). It seems that nine per cent of all spending on toys is by adults buying playthings for themselves as 'an escape from the stresses and strains of modern-day living' (ibid.) and using play as a means of connecting with other people in a world beset by loneliness. However, on the same day as we read of adults staking their claim to play, the BBC also reported the results of a survey by The Children's Society which found that 22 per cent of young people in the UK have self-harmed (Therrien 2018). The evidence is undeniable: if we want a society in which everyone has an equal chance of a happy and healthy life, we need to nurture the 'rebirth' of the spirit of play in society which was advocated by play pioneer, Dr Henry Curtis, over 100 years ago (Curtis 1917).

There is an ongoing discourse regarding the differential definitions of 'play' and 'playfulness' (Bateson and Martin 2013) which resonates throughout the book. The word 'play' has been used in the widely accepted sense to refer to the heterogeneous manifestations of self-motivated behaviors which are personally rewarding and which 'feel good' – which are fun (Bateson 2014). This definition embraces both the spontaneous, repetitive practice of novel behaviors common to all young mammals (Gray 2013) and the deep play of art and ritual (Ackerman 2000). Play is recognizable in that it 'looks different' (Bateson 2014) from other behaviors and activities. The word 'playfulness' (Bateson's 'playful play'; ibid.), used in the context of a typically 'non-play' behavior or situation, is used to refer to the application of a light-hearted disposition and a spontaneous willingness or inclination to deviate from social expectation so as to positively transform the meaning of an activity or situation. Thus, a serious health message (Chapter 3), a family meal (Chapter 7), or academic research (Chapter 11) can be labelled 'playful' when it shares play's central tenets of voluntary participation, engagement with process over outcome, and the generation of positive feeling. Throughout this book, the terms 'play' and 'playfulness' are frequently used together to refer both to recognizable 'play' behaviors and to what are traditionally non-play activities undertaken with a playful disposition. In some chapters, the contributing author has refined or expanded the definition of 'play' or 'playfulness' to suit the chapter content.

It is the hope of the editors that this book will have a broad appeal, reaching a general readership as well as readers from relevant professional groups – both practitioners and policy-makers. The following chapters may be read sequentially, tracing the application of play across scientific, creative and social dimensions, but each chapter also stands alone and may be read selectively, according to individual reader interests.

Chapter 1 introduces the pursuit of public health through play and playfulness, exploring how the science and the art of public health can interact with what is now known about the importance of play from cradle to grave.

Chapter 2 dissects the playful brain, exposing how play as an evolutionary mechanism impacts on mental capital through the life-course.

Chapter 3 explores the science of public health, highlighting how play and playfulness can contribute to the three pillars of protection, promotion and prevention.

Chapter 4 presents the contrasting perspective of artistic and creative endeavor as a route to public health, acknowledging the historical and social importance of the relationship between the arts and human health and wellbeing.

Chapter 5 identifies the importance of relationships to the public health agenda and examines how the connections between individuals, families and their wider social networks need to accommodate opportunities for play and playfulness.

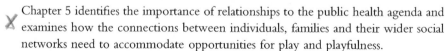

Chapter 6 debates the association between early attachment and the development of empathy. The chapter presents evidence to support the role of play as a mediator in this process and makes the case for play as a protective defence against the impact of adverse childhood experiences.

Chapter 7 examines how play can be used to mitigate against the pressures of modern family life. The chapter highlights the significance of family cohesion for public health and offers examples of the benefits of becoming a playful family.

Chapter 8 discusses how play and playfulness contribute to the public health agenda for children and adolescents, acknowledging the central role of play for helping children to reach their full potential.

Chapter 9 acknowledges the responsibility of public health for ensuring that the benefits of play can be accessed by all members of society. It recognizes societal barriers to playful participation and explores how creative innovation can help to overcome them.

Chapter 10 recognizes that the benefits of play can be carried forward into the workplace, enhancing productivity, creativity, and the health and wellbeing of the workforce. The chapter concludes by exploring how play and playfulness contributes to health and wellbeing beyond the working years.

Chapter 11 challenges the perception of digital play as purely a means of entertainment and embraces the notion that digital play can also be used as a facilitator of personal and professional engagement with public health.

Chapter 12 examines the concept of the playful setting as it links to the public health agenda, contrasting the play opportunities found within both natural and built environments.

Chapter 13 explores how the intervention of the state is necessary to facilitate playful strategies that can promote and protect the health of the population.

Chapter 14 concludes the book and presents the challenging concept of the application of play at the end of life. Contemporary approaches to death and dying are becoming increasingly 'playful', reflecting a public readiness to confront a final public health taboo.

We live in an era of global disillusionment with the socio-political status quo (Wike et al. 2016) yet there remains a collective belief in the power of ordinary citizens to drive change, whether in terms of child wellbeing (e.g. Save Childhood Movement, www.savechildhood.net), gender equality (e.g. #genderequality on Twitter), or ecological preservation (e.g. Plastic Pollution Coalition, www.plasticp ollutioncoalition.org). We find ourselves in an era of 'people power', where change comes about not so much by government diktat but through the will – the goodwill – of the people. Witness the rapid rise of the #MeToo movement (Khomami 2017) and Change.org, 'the fastest growing website for social change in the world' (Change.org 2018). Duncombe (2012) writes that 'to be a realist, you need to take dreams seriously'. In our play we are free to dream and it is the business of public health to make those dreams a reality.

In Benjamin Shepard's 2011 book, *Play, Creativity, and Social Movements: If I Can't Dance, It's Not My Revolution,* he argues that, in order to achieve change, we need to 'step away from stark reality to conjure up new possibilities for the present and our common future' (Shepard 2011: 46). The stark reality of public health in the 21st century is that there are huge social disparities in morbidity and mortality rates. In the UK we are fatter (Darzi 2018), less fit (Public Health England 2018), and more stressed (Mental Health Foundation 2018) than at any previous period in our history. We have an aging population and our health and social care systems are under ever-increasing pressure from raised demand and expectation. Bateson (2014) proposes that 'coming up with new ideas requires a different mindset from usefully implementing a new idea' and this applies to the arena of public health as much as to any other aspect of life. The time is ripe for the 'conjuring of new possibilities', for us to take bold steps towards more creative solutions and to re-examine the potential of play and playfulness for achieving change which is based on a publicly endorsed 'culture of health'.

## References

Ackerman, D. (2000) *Deep Play*, New York: Vintage Books.

Bateson, P. (2014) Playfulness and Creativity, *Animal Behavior and Cognition*, 1(2): 99–112.

Bateson, P. and Martin, P. (2013) *Play, Playfulness, Creativity and Innovation*, Cambridge: Cambridge University Press.

Brown, S. (2008) Play is More Than Just Fun, retrieved from www.ted.com/talks/stuart_brown_says_play_is_more_than_fun_it_s_vital (accessed 4 September 2018).

Change.org (2018) The World's Platform for Change, retrieved from www.change.org/l/uk/p/press (accessed 3 September 2018).

Curtis, H. S. (1917) *The Play Movement and its Significance*, New York: The Macmillan Company.

Darzi, A. (2018) Obesity Epidemic Demands More Action and Investment to Protect Children, retrieved from www.theguardian.com/theobserver/2018/jun/24/obesity-crisis-demands-more-action-and-investment (accessed 13 July 2018).

Duncombe, S. (2012) Book Review: Benjamin Shepard, Play, Creativity, and Social Movements: If I Can't Dance, It's Not My Revolution, *International Journal of Communication*, 6: 295–297.

Gray, P. (2013) Play as Preparation for Learning and Life. An Interview with Peter Gray, *American Journal of Play*, 5(3): 271–292.

Kane, P. (2012) Play and Lifestyle: State of 'The Play Ethic' 2012: interview with Viewpoint magazine, retrieved from www.theplayethic.com/playlifestyle_ch_5 (accessed 3 September 2018).

Khomami, N. (2017) #MeToo: How a Hashtag Became a Rallying Cry against Sexual Harassment, retrieved from www.theguardian.com/world/2017/oct/20/women-worldwide-use-hashtag-metoo-against-sexual-harassment (accessed 3 September 2018).

Mental Health Foundation (2018) Mental Health Statistics: Stress, retrieved from www.mentalhealth.org.uk/statistics/mental-health-statistics-stress (accessed 13 July 2018).

Peachey, K. (2018) Age: 43. Hobby: Lego. Rise of the Middle-Aged Toy Fans, retrieved from www.bbc.co.uk/news/business-45247637 (accessed 3 September 2018).

Public Health England (2018) Physical Activity Data Tool: Statistical Commentary, April 2018, retrieved from www.gov.uk/government/publications/physical-activity-data-tool-april-2018-update/physical-activity-data-tool-statistical-commentary-april-2018 (accessed 13 July 2018).

Shepard, B. (2011) *Play, Creativity, and Social Movements: If I Can't Dance, It's Not My Revolution*, New York: Routledge.

Therrien, A. (2018) Fifth of 14-Year-Old Girls in UK 'Have Self-Harmed', retrieved from www.bbc.co.uk/news/health-45329030 (accessed 3 September 2018).

Whitebread, D. with Basilio, M., Kuvalja, M. and Verma, M. (2012) *The Importance of Play*, Brussels: Toy Industries of Europe.

Wike, R., Fetterolf, J. and Parker, B. (2016) Even in Era of Disillusionment, Many Around the World Say Ordinary Citizens Can Influence Government, retrieved from www.pew global.org/2016/10/24/even-in-era-of-disillusionment-many-around-the-world-sa y-ordinary-citizens-can-influence-government (accessed 13 July 2018).

Yogman, M., Garner, A., HutchinsonJ., Hirsh-Pasek, K., Michnick Golinkoff, R. and Committee on Psychosocial Aspects of Child and Family Health, Council on Communications and Media (2018) The Power of Play: A Pediatric Role in Enhancing Development in Young Children, *Pediatrics*, 142(3): 1–16.

# 1

# IMPROVING THE PUBLIC'S HEALTH THROUGH PLAYFUL ENDEAVORS

*Julia Whitaker and Alison Tonkin*

## Introduction

Health is widely regarded as one of the most precious values in life, and the pursuit of health is a highly valued endeavor in both personal and public domains. Most developed regions, including the US, Canada, Western and Central Europe, as well as Nordic countries, rate health (along with life satisfaction) as what matters most to them in life (New Point de View 2015). A healthy life has become synonymous with life itself since, without some degree of healthy functionality, the living whole ceases to exist (Watt 2015). The relationship between a society's economic, social, and political stability and the health of its citizens is widely recognized as a main determinant of its success (Stoever and Kim 2007).

In 2014, the National Health Service in the UK published a 'Five Year Forward Review' which highlights the central role of public health in achieving societal goals, by engaging people and communities as active players in the search for new ways of addressing health concerns (NHS England 2014). Health has become a 'social movement', marking a shift from formal to informal approaches to health improvement in 'a persevering people-powered effort' (del Castillo et al. 2016: 9) to find creative solutions to current health challenges.

A parallel social movement has arisen from the study of play and playfulness (Shephard 2013). Playfulness is widely recognized as an innate human trait crucial for interpreting the world and responsible for engendering the creativity of thought and behavior which allows for adaptation to its constantly changing circumstances (de Koven 2017). While playfulness is widely encouraged in childhood, with designated space, time and encouragement for play, permission for adults to play tends to be limited to specific circumstances and is usually associated with purposeful activity (Rogerson et al. 2013). However, the fact that humans have developed a wide range of spontaneous play behaviors 'from doodling when bored to risky adventure play'

(Graham and Burghardt 2010: 403) suggests a significant function of playfulness in adulthood. A popular explanation for the continuation of play through the lifespan is that it supports the development of complex cognition and behavioral flexibility. Research into adult play acknowledges playfulness to be a variable which 'enables people to transform a situation or an environment in a way to allow for enjoyment or entertainment' (Proyer 2012: 1).

It is the transformational power of play and playfulness which now invites its serious consideration in the exploration of innovative approaches to the public health challenges of the 21st century. Recognizing the potential role of playfulness in relation to health demands a cultural shift from a 'top down' approach to one in which citizens can explore a new kind of creative freedom (Shephard 2013). Hannah asserts that the process of change 'starts by planting seeds of the new culture in the soil of the old' (Hannah 2014: 132): the playful pursuit of public health represents an attempt to add seeds of enjoyment and fun to the diverse mix of transformational possibilities.

## Defining public health

Public health is a concept which represents society's efforts to 'improve the health of the population and prevent illness' (Nuffield Council on Bioethics 2007: v). The emphasis on society means that, unlike medicine which focuses on the diagnosis, treatment and promotion of the health of an individual, public health requires society as a whole to embrace and engage, at local, national and international levels, with resources intended to provide the necessary conditions to live a healthy life (Chavan 2016).

With a rich and varied history, the concept of public health stretches back over ten thousand years to a time when nomadic lifestyles were replaced by a more communal and settled style of living (Science Museum n.d.). Societal change brought with it new challenges as contact between people, animals, and their associated waste products increased. Polluted water and the absence of appropriate waste disposal systems were responsible for the spread of disease and there was a growing recognition that this could be addressed through simple adaptations to this new way of life. Although there was little understanding of what contributed to the promotion of good health or the causes of disease, 'health' became a concept of communal concern leading to the emergence of a public approach to the health of the population (Science Museum n.d.).

The first recognized definition of public health practice was composed by Winslow in 1920. Nearly 70 years later, this was abbreviated and subsequently adopted by the World Health Organization (WHO), who define public health as 'The science and art of preventing disease, prolonging life and promoting health through the organized efforts of society' (Acheson, cited in WHO Regional Office for Europe 2017).

This definition reflects the importance of a dual approach to public health that relies on science to provide the surveillance, evidence base, and research capability to help people stay healthy and prevent ill health (Public Health England 2017) combined with the 'art of public persuasion' (Canadian Medical Association Journal

2000) which is needed to engage the public as active partners, enabling them to play their part in securing their own health and wellbeing wherever possible.

Modern public health practice necessitates partnership-working between everyone who contributes to the health of the population, acknowledging the multifaceted nature of health (Faculty of Public Health 2010). Many of the determinants of health and wellbeing that influence this are captured by Barton (2017) in Figure 1.1 which specifically recognizes the important contribution made by play. It also clearly identifies that policy and the role of the state are fundamental influences on public health, shaping the social circumstances of our lives, the communities we live in, and ultimately the choices we make when addressing risk factors to our health and wellbeing (Public Health England 2016).

The significance of play is also acknowledged by the American Public Health Association (2017), who state that 'Public health promotes and protects the health of people and the communities where they live, learn, work and play'. Within this definition, play is identified as a unitary aspect of the life of the community, making play a worthy concept to explore in the context of pursuing public health. Play takes many forms (Sutton-Smith 1980) and it is 'the richness and variety of our human games which make for a healthy and vibrant culture' (Kane 2004:7). A synthesis of the insights about the nature and function of play, provided by both the natural and the social sciences, opens-up the debate about the place of play in contemporary society (Kane 2004).

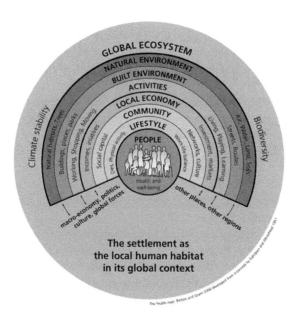

**FIGURE 1.1** The Settlement Health Model.
Source: Barton (2017); reproduced by kind permission of Professor Hugh Barton, University of the West of England

Nevertheless, play as a unitary concept is contentious: Gauntlett et al. (2010: 46) note that 'the world is still far from sharing a single view on the role or value of play in society'. Advocating play as a means of facilitating public health may be antagonistic but this does not preclude exploration of its status as a potentially low cost, high impact, and enjoyable means of engaging and enabling society's contribution to the public health agenda.

## Defining play

Definitions of play embedded in both the academic literature and in common parlance have provocatively incorporated elements of both the empirical and the philosophical, the rational and the esoteric. Play is explained as an innate drive, essential to mammalian survival and development (Koch 2017), yet widely recognized to be a voluntary activity (Garvey 1990) which is freely chosen (Hughes 2012) and culturally determined (Gosso and Almeida Carvalho 2013). The paradox of play (McCarthy 2007) revolves on the apparent contradiction that play is deemed essential to healthy growth and development (Ginsberg 2007) while simultaneously representing an exercise of personal free will (Baggini 2015).

In his classic text *Homo Ludens*, Huizinga (1949) identifies 'free choice' as the first main characteristic of play, differentiating it from all other aspects of natural or cultural life. Play is, perhaps, our only 'optional' pursuit, having neither specified purpose nor pre-determined ending (Gadamer 2013[1960]). The free nature of play is complemented by its identification with something *out-of-the-ordinary*, detached from everyday life yet integral to it; 'a necessity both for the individual … and for society by reason of the meaning it contains, its significance, its expressive value, its spiritual and social associations' (Huizinga 1949: 9). Play transfers and transforms the meanings attributed to the mundane and, in so doing, has the power to create the world anew (McCarthy 2007).

Contemporary research endorses 'freedom to play' as essential to the development of positive health and wellbeing, as well as to social and ecological survival (Gray 2009). Play is known to have a significant role in physiological development (Trawick-Smith 2014); in the maturation of social and communication skills (Goldstein 2012); and in creativity and problem solving (Brown 2008). There is also robust support for its role in the development of the flexible and non-specialist behaviors necessary for survival in a constantly changing ecological and cultural context (Pellegrini, 2009). The flexibility of movement, thought and behavior that are characteristic of play correspond to an adaptability to change that is essential for the evolution of strong and healthy communities (Sutton-Smith 1997).

## Free to play

The notion of *freedom* is encapsulated in the language used to describe play throughout history and across cultures. *Freedom of movement* is the concrete starting point for many play words (Huizinga 1949), whether referring to the movement of the wind and waves (the Sanskrit *krīdati*); the frolicking of young children and animals (the Greek *paidia*); or lively self-expression through dance and drama (the High German *leich*, the Anglo-Saxon *lâcan*). Yet the freedom integral to the concept of play goes beyond its allusion to freedom of physical movement: it also infers freedom of thought, behavior and opinion (the Latin *ludere,* meaning to twist words; the Chinese *wan,* referring to jesting or mockery). Perhaps most relevant to our consideration of play as it relates to the health of the social group, is the Indo-European root of the Old-English word *plegian* (also common to Celtic, German, Slavic and possibly Latin), namely the word *dlegh* meaning 'to engage oneself' (Kane 2004). Play is essentially a social activity (McLean and Hurd 2014), a means of 'engaging oneself' with the external world, with others, and with different parts of the self. It is the complex interplay between social engagement and the health of individuals and communities (Bennett 2005) which reinforces the role for play in the public health debate.

All social activities come about in relation to cultural narratives and their embedded practices, and the notion of engaging, or indulging oneself, with the freedom of movement, thought and behavior that is play has influenced the popular perception of play throughout history.

## The historical evolution of play as a means of social engagement

The nature of play has preoccupied scholars since the time of the ancient Greeks. Plato wrote in *The Republic* (*c.*360 BCE: Waterfield 1993) of the importance of freedom, for learning and for understanding the human condition (Frost et al. 2012). Elements of play were intrinsic to a range of cultural activities in Ancient Greece (500–323 BCE): the playing of games and music featured in both ceremonial and social gatherings, and drinking parties included the exchange of verses and riddles. In the agrarian context of Greek society, intellectual discourse was regarded as much a playful alternative to work as the display of athletic and sporting prowess (D'Angour 2013). The Greek concepts of *agon* (contest), *mimesis* (symbolic depiction) and *chaos* (chance and fate) remain constants in contemporary attempts to create a framework for understanding the play concept (Sutton-Smith 1997).

History reveals the positive and valuable contribution of play to the socialization of humans as a species, particularly as they congregated into larger communal groups. However, it is also the case that related changes in lifestyle and behavior were accompanied by detrimental consequences to health and wellbeing. The impact of indulgent behaviors is believed to predate the times of the ancient Greeks: the Venus figurines dating from 35,000 to 20,000 BCE are 'believed to be the first sculptural representations of the human body … and some are astonishingly corpulent-huge [with] pendulous breasts, gigantic bellies, and enormous thighs' (Dossey 2010: 3). Many believe that these figurines are actual representations of the human form of that period and that they depict mass obesity (ibid.). Challenging the perception that obesity is a modern phenomenon, the portrayal of obesity dates back to the Palaeolithic era and reappears in the European art of the Renaissance period. In early Christian European art, only those from low socio-economic backgrounds were portrayed as obese while in Greek and Roman art corpulence is conspicuously absent, reflecting the ideals of society at the time, certainly for the Greeks who extolled the virtues of moderation in the quest for the 'ideal human' (ibid.).

Social life in Ancient Rome (753 BCE–476 CE) was clearly divided between work (*negotium*) and leisure (*otium*). Popular leisure activities included social play aspects such as swimming, athletics and theatrical performance. The public bathhouse (the Roman 'leisure centre') was a social space devoted to relaxation, and often contained a courtyard (*palaestra*) used for exercise, a library, lecture hall, gymnasium, and formal gardens (Fife 2012).

The Romans are generally recognized as having established the first-ever system of public health. They understood the association between health and hygiene and provided facilities – such as public baths, sewers and toilets – to promote public health. They needed these measures to maintain the health of their military forces as they strove to keep their growing empire under control (BBC 2014). However, despite good intentions and the desire to create a healthier society, archaeological findings suggest that public health may actually have suffered as a result of Roman innovation (Kennedy 2016). The Romans spread disease and pestilence across the Empire, evidenced through skeletal and cesspit remains, as well as artefacts such as fine combs for removing lice and other parasites. Roman physicians recognized that parasites caused disease but their prescribed remedies, such as the use of hot water and bloodletting, actually made things worse (ibid.).

The decline of the Roman Empire in the East is believed to have been accelerated by the spread of bubonic plague, transmitted by fleas, in the 6th century (Kennedy 2016). Although much of the Roman public health infrastructure was lost with the decline of the Roman Empire, the subsequent rise of an Islamic Empire was accompanied by innovative healthcare facilities and public health arrangements, with many cities boasting sewage systems and public baths (Science Museum n.d.).

The Viking age (800 CE–1066 CE) heralded a new era of play-related activity, illustrating the contribution made by play and playfulness to the integration of cultural variance as new societal groupings emerge. The multi-faceted nature of play is supported by archaeological evidence from the period. Play as contest was enacted both in vigorous outdoor games based on warrior skills and in competitive board games such as *Hnefatafl*, a precursor to chess. Social play in the form of drinking games which involved the exchange of boasts, insults and mockery, was a popular pastime along with singing and storytelling. Viking children mimicked adult play in child versions of adult games and in the imitation of aspects of community life (Hurstwic 2017).

These historical accounts of early social play reveal it to be firstly an adult initiative: the play behavior of the young chiefly an imitation or representation of the observed activities of their elders. Social playfulness would seem to be critical to both the cultural welfare and to the evolution of the group (Panksepp 2015). Ancient history offers a perception of play as a positive feature of inter-generational social and cultural life, celebrated publicly and across social groupings. However, the free nature of play and the challenge it poses to established thought and behavior was set to confront the purposeful work ethic and the devaluing of playful pursuits which accompanied the rise and spread of Early Christianity (Kane 2004).

In anticipation of the end of the world with the Second Coming of Jesus Christ, early Christians placed great emphasis on the purposeful use of time, and 'idleness' was re-categorized as sinful by the church fathers who condemned the hedonism of their pagan antecedents (Hill 1999). The prevalence of pestilence, plague and disease which blighted the medieval period, together with renewed urbanization in Eastern Europe, prompted the spread of a fanatical asceticism throughout the Eastern Roman Empire and contributed to the widening appeal of the monastic life. A general disdain for plea-sure-seeking marked a social shift in the perception of play which was to be reflected in the rise of the *Protestant work ethic*, which has pervaded many Christian cultures since the Reformation of the Church in the Middle Ages (McLean and Hurd 2014).

Popular contempt for the role of 'political interference' in matters of public health may be linked back to this era. Religious scorn for indulgence meant that behaviors linked to the consumption of food and alcohol and sexual behavior became stigmatized (Science Museum n.d.) and moral regulation for the 'benefit' of society was aggressively pursued. The Church fathers used fear to impose social control through reference to scripture which supported the disdain of pleasure and indulgence (Unger and Scherer 2010).

The crossing of the Atlantic by early European settlers witnessed the trans-portation of their Puritan contempt for all things pleasurable to the New World. The playful behaviors of indigenous tribes were regarded with both intrigue and suspicion by the incomers, because of their perceived 'purposelessness' (Dyson 2015). Increasing prosperity was subsequently accompanied by the introduction of sanctioned amusements, but these were clearly defined, 'purposeful' activities typically associated with civic occasions and agricultural fairs.

Kaiser (2012) attributes the modern concept of play as a way of making meaning in the world to the Victorians, who bequeathed us *Alice in Wonderland*, the pre-Raphaelites and Dickens – as well as Christmas, the seaside, public parks and the weekend. Play is now recognized as a way of simultaneously assuming agency and of letting go, a 'mutation of real conflicts and functions … always intended to serve a healing function' (Sutton-Smith 2015). Linking play to the public health agenda is about unleashing its potential as a 'game-changer' in the pursuit of a new approach to the challenging complexities of health provision in the current social and economic context.

## Linking play to public health

The potency of play is enhanced when undertaken as a social activity and, as noted in the historical context above, there is an overlap between the concepts of public health and play. The need for human connection supports the founding principles of public health, and playful endeavors provide the perfect vehicle to facilitate society's response to current concerns about the health of the population. Hannah (2014:4) suggests that 'Health is a product of healthy relationships, a quality of life held in common … that nobody can be healthy alone'.

Play complements the defined duality of public health, providing a unifying con-cept by virtue of play being 'an essential process in artistic and scientific creativity'

(Schore 2017). This duality is reflected in how our brain operates, each brain hemisphere producing a unique set of associated personality traits (Miller 2012), as shown in Figure 1.2. The advertising industry has long exploited the science behind personality typology for commercial gain and public health could usefully borrow from this targeted approach to public engagement. It suggests that a multilayer approach, which utilizes a range of engagement strategies and activities, will be needed if all elements of society are to be taken into consideration.

The remainder of this chapter will explore in more detail the potential contribution of play and playfulness to the scientific and artistic pursuit of public health, with particular reference to how this may help to organize and enhance society's contribution to the public health agenda.

## The science of public health

Scientific discovery provides the foundation of the modern public health movement, dating back to the growing interest in the trends and patterns of disease proliferation in the early 18th century.

> Counting and valuing – characteristics of trading nations with growing empires – were now applied to populations. Censuses, disease statistics, birth rates and bills of mortality marked the earliest beginnings of epidemiology, the 'science' of public health.
>
> *(Science Museum n.d.)*

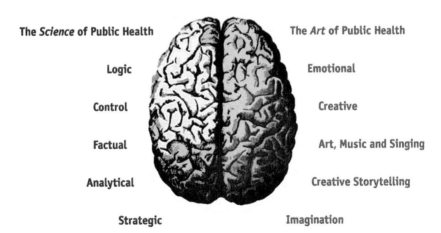

**FIGURE 1.2** Personality traits linked to public health that are associated with the two hemispheres of the brain.
Source: Annette Gossett (adapted from Miller 2012)

Epidemiology is a central component of the public health system and in the latest strategic planning undertaken by Public Health England (2016: 16) epidemiology is tasked to: 'strengthen our capacities in emergency preparedness, resilience and response to ensure seamless connections between local, national and global responses'.

One example of how epidemiology can be applied to public health, is in relation to the factors that contribute to premature death. Kirkwood (cited Cayton 2001) notes that, genetically, we are not programmed to die and that, theoretically, the frailties of old age are a consequence of systems failure as a result of disease and ill health. Public Health England (2016) has identified a range of factors that contribute to premature death as shown in Figure 1.3, and it is worth noting that only 10 per cent is linked to the provision of healthcare.

Hannah (2014) suggests that we already possess infinite human resources with the potential to positively influence our health: the potential for playful endeavors is indicated in 95 per cent of the areas identified in Figure 1.3 and summarized below:

- Genetic predisposition (30 per cent): We are genetically predisposed to play (Brown and Vaughan 2009) but society needs to provide opportunities and permission to play through the life course and the political will to enable this to happen.
- Behavioral patterns (40 per cent): We adopt behavioral patterns from an early age, but as a species we are adaptable, changeable, and can acquire and build new skills through brain plasticity. Dolan et al. (2010) suggest that using emotional cues at an unconscious level and appealing to the right side of our brain is an area worthy of exploration – the art of public persuasion using

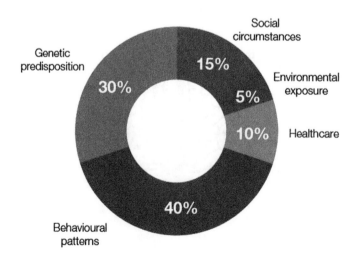

**FIGURE 1.3** Proportional contribution to premature death.
Source: Public Health England (2016: 7); Open Government Licence 3.0 (www. nationalarchives.gov.uk/doc/open-government-licence/version/3)

behavioral politics is an emerging science and playful endeavors can provide a
means of facilitating this.

- Social circumstances (15 per cent): These shape the choices we make and contribute
  to a range of risk factors that influence our health and wellbeing both as individuals
  and society as a whole (Public Health England 2016). Play is reflected throughout
  the environment in which we work, live and are educated, which links back to the
  definition of public health by the American Public Health Association (2017).
- Healthcare (10 per cent): Art in healthcare has been used for centuries, but art
  is now increasingly being recognized as a means of preventing disease and
  improving wellbeing (National Alliance for Arts, Health and Wellbeing 2017).
  Art can enhance the environment, encourage participation, and is used for
  education and training as well as a means of therapy.

## The art of public health

Like play, health and healing are organic processes characterized by their uncertain
outcomes (Panda 2006). Health is a nebulous concept, the meaning of which is
dependent on the exercise of practical judgement and personal interpretation (Gadamer
1996). There has long been an understanding that, just as the health of the individual is
more than simply a question of biology, the health of society cannot be understood in
socio-political terms alone. Throughout history, the personal and societal interpretation
of health has been reflected in artistic representations of the human body and this has
varied across time and culture (Dossey 2010). There are many examples of the use of
visual imagery to explore both personal experiences and public perceptions of health
and illness (Harrison 2002). From sexually explicit fertility symbols of the Palaeolithic
era (Nature Video n.d.) to Leonardo da Vinci's precise anatomical drawings, and from
the 18th-century poem 'The Art of Preserving Health' (Budd 2016) to Sigga Ella's
photographic profiles of people with Down's syndrome (Ella 2016), art has enlivened
and enriched perceptions of health and its place in public consciousness.

At every level, the delivery, nurturance and recovery of positive health is concerned
with connection: with the parts of the self, with the social group, and with nature
(Zeedyk 2018). The creation of connections which foster health and healing requires
the same expression or application of human creativity and imagination required of the
painter, sculptor, or musician. The 'art' of public health, therefore, involves engaging
both the designated 'healers' in our society and their subjects in the co-creation of
connective systems and processes which reflect the human qualities of kindness,
compassion and solidarity (Heath 2017) and which reinforce the potential for
resilience in the face of adversity.

## Conclusion

There is a risk that, in an attempt to grant legitimacy to the serious exploration of
play as a healthful concept, we feel compelled to accommodate to the predominating
bio-mechanical model of what constitutes positive health (Marcum 2004). In our

efforts to justify the worth of play and playfulness in relation to standard measures of health, we adopt the language of scientific methodology to demonstrate their clinical and economic benefits: play is described as an 'intervention' or 'strategy' with 'out-comes' which can be subjected to scientific 'evaluation' (Li et al. 2016). Sharing a common language may facilitate the communication of ideas but 'shared commit-ment only comes after shared understanding' (Thomas and McDonagh 2013), which in turn depends on openness, mutual respect, and a shared intent.

Hannah (2014) challenges us to acknowledge the limits of 'mechanistic thinking' in the ongoing search for a new model of healthcare which is better suited to the complexities of contemporary health concerns in the current social and economic context. A recognition of play as central to this 'new model' of health invites expla-nation but no apology: play in the context of public health represents an opportunity to integrate the latest scientific insights into brain function and development with the humanistic qualities of humility, curiosity and connectivity (Chou et al. 2014). Hui-zinga (1949) writes of the 'agonistic' qualities of play in its challenge to existing viewpoints in the public sphere. The proposal that play might have something important to contribute to the current public health agenda critiques prevailing reductive approaches but need not totally undermine them. Chambers (2001) clarifies that 'an agonistic discourse will … be one marked not merely by conflict but just as importantly, by mutual admiration …'.

The study and practice of play are both *science* and *art*. Research in the field of neuro-science reveals the changes in brain function and process which occur as a result of play and which are manifest in 'more useful social strategies and more flexible behavioral responses to unexpected future events' (Panksepp 2010). The 'art' of play is represented in the countless imaginative possibilities for creating relation-ships, systems and environments that are more conducive to these more healthful attitudes and behaviors. In his manifesto for a *play ethic*, Kane (2004: 11) writes:

> Much of the benefit of play … is that it helps us to make reality amenable to our will. It renders the real virtual and gives us the chance, through our games and simulations, to test out our future options.

In advocating for a 'playful' pursuit of public health, this book integrates the evidence from scientific and creative endeavors to support a *third way* (International Futures Forum 2017) towards improved health and wellbeing from cradle to grave.

## References

American Public Health Association (2017) What is Public Health?, retrieved from www.ap ha.org/what-is-public-health (accessed 3 September 2018).
Baggini, J. (2015) *Freedom Regained: The Possibility of Free Will*, London: Granta.
Barton, H. (2017) *City of Well-being: A Radical Guide to Planning*, Abingdon: Routledge.
BBC (2014) Roman Public Health, retrieved from www.bbc.co.uk/schools/gcsebitesize/his tory/shp/ancient/romanpublichealthrev1.shtml (accessed 6 July 2017).

Bennett, K. (2005) Social Engagement as a Longitudinal Predictor of Objective and Subjective Health, *European Journal of Ageing*, 2: 48–55.

Brown, S. (2008) Play Is More Than Just Fun, retrieved from www.ted.com/talks/stuart_brown_says_play_is_more_than_fun_it_s_vital/transcript?language=en#t-1347443 (accessed 6 June 2017).

Brown, S. and Vaughan, C. (2009) *Play: How It Shapes the Brain, Opens the Imagination, and Invigorates the Soul*, New York: Avery.

Budd, A. (2016) *John Armstrong's The Art of Preserving Health: Eighteenth-Century Sensibility in Practice*, London: Routledge.

Canadian Medical Association Journal (2000) Editorial: Public Health, Public Persuasion, *Canadian Medical Association Journal*, 162(7): 961.

Cayton, H. (2001) From Childhood to Childhood? Autonomy, Dignity and Dependence through the Ages of Life, 15th Alzheimer's Disease International Conference, Christchurch, New Zealand, October.

Chambers, S. (2001) Language and Politics: Agonistic Discourse in The West Wing, retrieved from www.ctheory.net/articles.aspx?id=317 (accessed 28 June 2017).

Chavan, M. (2016) What is Public Health?, retrieved from www.medicalhealthscience.com/2016/11/what-is-public-health-p-ublichealth-is.html (accessed 14 June 2017).

Chou, C., Kellom, K. and Shea, J. (2014) Attitudes and Habits of Highly Humanistic Physicians, *Academic Medicine*, 89(9):1252–1258.

D'Angour, A. (2013) Plato and Play: Taking Education Seriously in Ancient Greece, *American Journal of Play*, 5(3): 293–307.

De Koven, B. (2017) Ten Paradoxical Traits of the Playful Personality, retrieved from www.deepfun.com/ten-paradoxical-traits-of-the-playful-personality (accessed 7 July 2017).

Del Castillo, J., Khan, H., Nicholas, L. and Finnis, A. (2016) *Health as a Social Movement: The Power of People in Movements*, London: Nesta.

Dolan, P.Hallsworth, M.Halpern, D.King, D. and Vlaev, I. (2010) *Mindspace: Influencing behaviour through Public Policy*, London: Institute for Government.

Dossey, L. (2010) Gluttony and Obesity, *Explore*, 6(1): 1–6.

Dyson, J. (2015) Play in America: A Historical Overview, in J. Johnson, S. Eberle, T. Henricks and D. Kuschner (eds), *The Handbook of the Study of Play, Vol 1*, 41–50, Baltimore, MD: Rowman & Littlefield.

Ella, S. (2016) First and Foremost I Am, retrieved from https://siggaella.com/projects/first-and-foremost-i-am (accessed 6 July 2017).

Faculty of Public Health (2010) What is Public Health?, retrieved from www.fph.org.uk/what_is_public_health (accessed 17 October 2016).

Fife, S. (2012) Athletics, Leisure, and Entertainment in Ancient Rome, retrieved from www.ancient.eu/article/98 (accessed 6 June 2017).

Frost, J., Wortham, S. and Reifel, S. (2012) *Play and Child Development*, 4th edition, Upper Saddle Riover, NJ: Pearson Education.

Gadamer, H.J. (2013[1960]) *Truth and Method*, London: Bloomsbury.

Gadamer, H.G. (1996) *The Enigma of Health: The Art of Healing in a Scientific Age*, Stanford, CA: Stanford University Press.

Garvey, C. (1990). *Play*, Cambridge, MA: Harvard University Press.

Gauntlett, D., Ackermann, E., Whitebread, D., Wolbers, T. and Weckstrom, C. (2010) *The Future of Play. Defining the Role and Value of Play in the 21st Century*, Billund, Denmark: LEGO Learning Institute.

Ginsberg, K. (2007) The Importance of Play in Promoting Healthy Child Development and Maintaining Strong Parent-Child Bonds, *Pediatrics*, 119(1): 182–191.

Goldstein, J., 2012, *Play in Children's Health, Development and Wellbeing*, Brussels: Toy Industries of Europe.

Gosso, Y. and Almeida Carvalho, M. (2013) Play and Cultural Context, retrieved from www.child-encyclopedia.com/sites/default/files/textes-experts/en/774/play-and-cultura l-context.pdf (accessed 21 June 2017).

Graham, K. and Burghardt, G. (2010) Current Perspectives on the Biological Study of Play: Signs of Progress, *Quarterly Review of Biology*, 85(4):393–418.

Gray, P. (2009) Play as a Foundation for Hunter-Gatherer Social Existence, *American Journal of Play*, Spring: 476–521.

Hannah, M. (2014) *Humanising Healthcare: Patterns of Hope for a System under Strain*, Fife: International Futures Forum.

Harrison, B. (2002) Seeing Health and Illness Worlds – Using Visual Methodologies in a Sociology of Health and Illness: A Methodological Review, *Sociology of Health & Illness*, 24(6): 856–872.

Heath, I. (2017) Performing Medicine at SaIL, retrieved from http://performingmedicine. com/project/performing-medicine-at-sail (accessed 26 June 2017).

Hill, S. (1999) Historical Context of Work Ethic, retrieved from http://workethic.coe.uga. edu/historypdf.pdf (accessed 22 June 2017).

Hughes, B. (2012) *Evolutionary Playwork and Reflective Analytic Practice*, 2nd edition, London: Routledge.

Huizinga, J. (1949) *Homo Ludens: A Study of the Play-Element in Culture*, London: Routledge & Kegan Paul.

Hurstwic (2017) Games and Sports in the Viking Age, retrieved from www.hurstwic.org/ history/articles/daily_living/text/games_and_sports.htm (accessed 6 June 2017).

International Futures Forum (2017) Three Horizons, retrieved from www.internationalfu turesforum.com/three-horizons (accessed 28 June 2017).

Kaiser, M. (2012) *The World in Play. Portraits of a Victorian Concept*, Stanford, CA: Stanford University Press.

Kane, P. (2004) *The Play Ethic: A Manifesto for a Different Way of Living*, Basingstoke: Macmillan.

Kennedy, M. (2016) What Did the Romans Ever Do for Us? Lice, Fleas and Bacterial Infections, *The Guardian*, 8 January, retrieved from www.theguardian.com/science/2016/ jan/08/flea-bitten-empire-roman-gifts-to-the-world-included-bacterial-infections (acces sed 3 September 2018).

Koch, S. N. (2017) Play: An Innate Brain System, retrieved from http://mybrainnotes. com/autism-adhd-play.html (accessed 21 June 2017).

Li, W., Oi Kwan Chung, J., Yan Ho, K.and Chau Kwok, B. (2016) Play Interventions to Reduce Anxiety and Negative Emotions in Hospitalized Children, *BMC Pediatrics*, 16(1): 1.

McCarthy, D. (2007) *A Manual of Dynamic Play Therapy: Helping Things Fall Apart, the Paradox of Play*, London: Jessica Kingsley.

McLean, D. and Hurd, A. (2014) *Kraus' Recreation and Leisure in Modern Society*, Burlington, MA: Jones & Bartlett.

Marcum, J. (2004) Biomechanical and Phenomenological Models of the Body, the Meaning of Illness and Quality of Care, *Medicine, Healthcare, and Philosophy*, 7(3): 311–320.

Miller, J. (2012) Are You a Right-Brain or a Left-Brain Marketer?, retrieved from http:// blog.marketo.com/2012/01/the-right-brain-vs-left-brain-of-marketers.html (accessed 25 June 2017).

National Alliance for Arts, Health and Wellbeing (2017) What is Arts in Health?, retrieved from www.artshealthandwellbeing.org.uk/what-is-arts-in-health (accessed 25 June 2017).

Nature Video (n.d.) Pre-historic Pin-Up, retrieved from www.youtube.com/watch?v= Y8noVoCsYGs&feature=youtu.be (accessed 7 July 2017).

New Point de View (2015) What Value is Most Important to People in Each Country?, retrieved from www.newpointdeview.com/pro-en/what-value-is-most-important-to-p eople-in-each-country (accessed 7 July 2017).

NHS England (2014) Five Year Forward View, retrieved from www.england.nhs.uk/wp -content/uploads/2014/10/5yfv-web.pdf (accessed 7 July 2017).

Nuffield Council on Bioethics (2007) *Public Health: Ethical Issues*, London: Nuffield Council on Bioethics.

Panda, S. (2006) Medicine: Science or Art? *Mens Sana Monographs*, 4(1): 127–138.

Panksepp, J. (2010) Science of the Brain as a Gateway to Understanding Play: An Interview with Jaak Panksepp, *American Journal of Play*, Winter: 245–277.

Panksepp, J. (2015) Give Play a Chance: The Psychobiology of PLAY and the Benefits of Social Playfulness, in J. Johnson, S. Eberle, T. Henricks and D. Kuschner (eds), *The Handbook of the Study of Play, Vol 1*, 477–488, Baltimore, MD: Rowman & Littlefield.

Pellegrini, A. (2009) *The Role of Play in Human Development*, Oxford: Oxford University Press.

Proyer, R. (2012) Development and Initial Assessment of a Short Measure for Adult Play-fulness: the SMAP, Personality and Individual Differences, retrieved from http://scottba rrykaufman.com/wp-content/uploads/2012/08/Proyer-2012.pdf (accessed 7 July 2017).

Public Health England (2016) *Strategic Plan for the Next Four Years: Better Outcomes by 2020*, London: Public Health England.

Public Health England (2017) Refocusing Public Health England, retrieved from www.gov. uk/government/news/refocusing-public-health-england (accessed 24 June 2017).

Rogerson, R., Treadaway, C., Lorimer, H., Billington, J. and Fyfe, H. (2013) *Permission to Play: Taking Play Seriously in Adulthood*, Swindon: AHRC.

Schore, A. (2017) Playing on the Right Side of the Brain, *American Journal of Play*, 9(2):105–142.

Science Museum (n.d.) Public Health, retrieved from www.sciencemuseum.org.uk/brought tolife/themes/publichealth (accessed 23 June 2017).

Shepard, B. (2011) *Play, Creativity, and Social Movements: If I Can't Dance, It's Not My Revo-lution*, London: Routledge.

Stoever, K. and Kim, A. (2007) Thinking Globally: Global Health as a Factor in Economic and Social Stability. Health Progress, retrieved from www.chausa.org/docs/default-source/health-progress/thinking-globally—global-health-as-a-factor-in-economic-and-so cial-stability-pdf.pdf?sfvrsn=0 (accessed 7 July 2017).

Sutton-Smith, B. (1980) *Play and Learning*, Hoboken, NJ: John Wiley & Sons.

Sutton-Smith, B. (1997) *The Ambiguity of Play*, Cambridge MA: Harvard University Press.

Sutton-Smith, B. (2015) Play Theory: A Personal Journey and New Thoughts, in J. John-son, S. Eberle, T. Henricks and D. Kuschner (eds), *The Handbook of the Study of Play, Vol 1*, 239–270, Baltimore, MD: Rowman & Littlefield.

Thomas, J. and McDonagh, D. (2013) Shared Language: Towards More Effective Com-munication, *The Australasian Medical Journal*, 6(1): 46–54.

Trawick-Smith, J. (2014) The Physical Play and Motor Development of Young Children: A Review of Literature and Implications for Practice, retrieved from www.easternct.edu/ cece/files/2014/06/BenefitsOfPlay_LitReview.pdf (accessed 1 July 2017).

Unger, R. and Scherer, P. (2010) Gluttony, Sloth and the Metabolic Syndrome: A Road-map to Lipotoxicity, *Trends in Endocrinology and Metabolism*, 21: 345–352.

Waterfield, R. (1993) *Republic*, Oxford: Oxford University Press.

Watt, H. (2015) Life and Health: A Value in Itself for Human Beings? *HEC Forum*, 27(3): 207–228.

WHO Regional Office for Europe (2017) Public Health Services, retrieved from www.euro. who.int/en/health-topics/Health-systems/public-health-services (accessed 14 June 2017).

Zeedyk, S. (2018) The Science of Connection, retrieved from http://connectedbaby.net/ the-science-of-connection (accessed 3 September 2018).

# 2

## PLAYING FOR A HEALTHY BRAIN

*Alison Tonkin*

### Introduction

The notion of public health rests on the collective will of society to work with one another to fulfil the collective responsibility for health and wellbeing (Faculty of Public Health 2018). Although this responsibility ultimately rests with national public health agencies and local authorities (Alzheimer's Society 2014), we can do much as individuals to implement interventions that are linked to the promotion of healthier behavior across the population. Our thoughts, feelings and behavior are mediated by the brain and according to Perry et al. (2000: 9), this 'allows us our humanity'. The characteristics that define us as human beings are intimately associated with how the brain develops and matures, and play makes a significant contribution to this process.

This chapter will explore how play facilitates healthy brain development and functioning, aligned to the concept of mental capital which is acquired in child-hood and adolescence and maintained and developed in adulthood until its decline in older age (Foresight Mental Capital and Wellbeing Project 2008). Essentially, the chapter suggests that the more we play, at any stage of life, the more the brain benefits from the experience, which is encapsulated in the following statement by Brown (2008): '*Nothing lights up the brain like play*'.

### Setting the scene

The concept of mental capital is defined as 'the totality of an individual's cognitive and emotional resources, including their cognitive capability, flexibility and efficiency of learning, emotional intelligence (e.g. empathy and social cognition), and resilience in the face of stress. The extent of an individual's resources reflects his/her basic endowment (genes and early biological programming), and their experiences and education, which take place throughout the lifecourse' (Kirkwood et al. 2008: 7). Together, these resources determine the quality of life experience and how effectively an individual will be able to contribute to society (ibid.).

In 2008, the Foresight Mental Capital and Wellbeing Project, which had been set up to 'inform the UK government and the private sector on how to achieve the best possible mental development and mental wellbeing for everyone in the UK', presented its findings in a series of reports. Several system maps were published (Foresight Mental Capital and Wellbeing Project 2008) as visual representations of the factors that affect mental capital and wellbeing. The system maps demonstrate the interrelated nature of these factors and how they impinge on the public health agenda.

For example, the conceptual overview of 'mental capital through life' refers to biology, people, culture and environment as key influences, with sleep, nutrition and exercise running as constants throughout (Foresight Mental Capital and Wellbeing Project 2008). Although responsibility for health and wellbeing is often promoted as resting with the individual, Figure 2.1 clearly demonstrates that this is difficult to achieve at an individual level and that public health has a duty to lead society's efforts, many of which mirror the findings of the mental capital and wellbeing project.

The trajectory of mental capital follows a similar pattern to that of brain development, rising in the early years, levelling off in adulthood, before gradually trailing off towards the end of the natural life span as the reserves built-up through the life-course are depleted (Kirkwood et al. 2008). The following exploration of the links between play and playfulness and the brain suggests a rationale for play's inclusion as a tool for facilitating mental capital and the wider public health agenda.

## Evolution of the playful brain

The brain is not a single 'homogeneous organ' but a highly complex system with integrated and inter-related regions (Icahn School of Medicine 2016). These regions, which have evolved over millions of years, have distinct roles and functions which develop in a sequential, hierarchical fashion (Britto 2014; Gauntlett et al. 2010; Perry et al. 2000), as shown in Figure 2.2.

Kapit et al. (2000: 108) propose that the brain has developed as 'three brains in one', reflecting its evolutionary pathway:

- Lower – reflexive/vegetative brain.
- Intermediate – emotional and instinctive brain.
- Higher – adaptive/skilled brain.

### The lower brain

The neurodevelopmental sequencing of the brain starts from the most basic, reg-ulatory regions situated in the brainstem (Perry et al. 2000). This incorporates the medulla and pons, which carry out many of the visceral and reflexive activities,

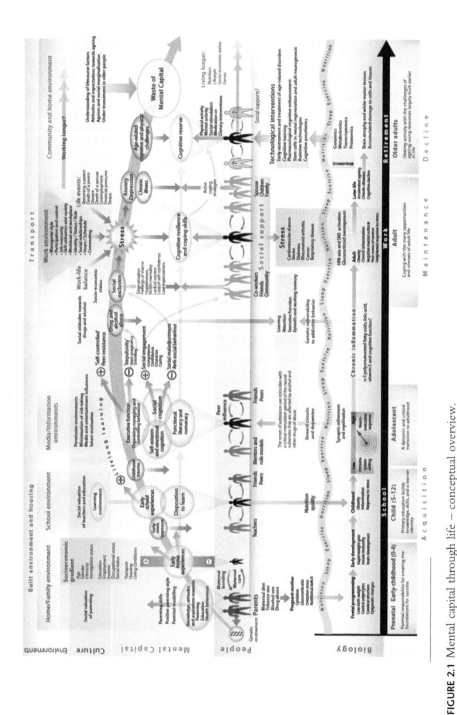

**FIGURE 2.1** Mental capital through life – conceptual overview.
Source: Foresight Mental Capital and Wellbeing Project (2008: 3); Open Government Licence 3.0 (www.nationalarchives.gov.uk/doc/open-government-licence/version/3)

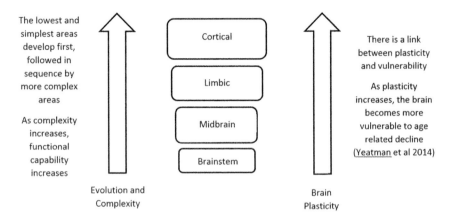

**FIGURE 2.2** Sequential neurodevelopment of the brain.
Source: adapted from Perry et al. (2000), cited in Child Trauma Academy (2002)

such as respiration, cardiovascular and digestive functioning (Kapit et al. 2000), as well as the regulation of sleep and fear states (Gooey Brains 2015). The midbrain, which is also considered to be part of the lower brain, regulates gross and fine motor skills and enables the integration of complex sensory information with other regions of the brain (ibid.). This 'lower brain' provides a stable base to which additional layers of complexity have been added over time (Yeatman et al. 2014).

## The intermediate brain

The limbic system consists of a set of structures that are located on both sides of the brain, including the hippocampus and the amygdala (Daffner 2016). The limbic system is 'responsible for emotions, values and other unique functions that control so much of human behavior' (Britto 2014). As this area of the brain develops, children gain skills associated with tolerance, empathy and emotional regulation, leading to an understanding of social relationships (Gooey Brains 2015; Brown and Vaughan 2009). Some of the limbic structures are also linked to the cognitive functions involved in memory processing (Kapit et al. 2000).

Over the course of mammalian evolution, there has been no significant change to the overall size and organization of the limbic system, suggesting that certain basic behaviors are common to all species of mammals (Kapit et al. 2000). This includes the playfulness exhibited by young mammals for whom play is a means of practising the skills needed to grow and to thrive and to reproduce in adulthood (Gray 2009). Gray (ibid.) goes on to suggest that 'we humans have inherited the basic youthful play characteristics of our animal ancestors, but in the course of our biological and cultural evolution we have elaborated upon them and created new functions'.

## *The higher brain*

The higher functions referred to by Gray (2009) have been made possible by the most recent evolutionary development – the cerebral cortex. Emerging above the lower centers, the cerebral cortex is made up of two non-identical cerebral hemispheres. They are not mirror images of each other and one hemisphere tends to dominate the other. Cortical mapping has identified four distinct lobes of the cerebral cortex, with the limbic system situated deep within these lobes (Kapit and Elson 1977). The 'higher brain' enables 'the highest and finest analysis of sensory and motor integration, learning and skilled tasks [which have become] the basis of adaptive capabilities, introspection, planning and speech in humans' (Kapit et al. 2000: 82). It also facilitates cognition and executive function, as well as consciousness and imagination, which have been instrumental in the emergence of collective concepts such as culture and the organization of society (Britto 2014).

Despite the distinct functionality of differing regions of the brain, even the simplest task involves simultaneous activity across multiple regions (Urban Child Institute 2016). This requires networks of specialized, excitable nerve cells called neurons to communicate with one another through electrical and chemical signals at connections called synapses (Urban Child Institute 2016). The human brain consists of tissue that can be divided into two categories: grey matter and white matter (Daffner 2016). The behavioral, cognitive, motor and sensory areas of the brain (grey matter) are connected by a mass of fibre pathways (white matter) which enable global functions such as learning, memory and consciousness (Kapit and Elson 1977). Grey matter forms the outer cerebral cortex with the characteristic deep grooves (fissures), hills (gyri), and furrows (sulci) which create the distinct contours of the brain (Kapit and Elson 1977). The underlying white matter consists of numerous tracts which act as a 'subway of the brain, connecting different regions of grey matter in the cerebrum to one another' (Balm 2014). White matter runs deep underneath grey matter enabling the transmission of electrical impulses due to myelination. Myelin sheaths encase 'each neuron's process transmitting signals to other neurons', insulating the electrical signals and enhancing the speed of transmission between neurons (ibid.).

At birth, the brain is technically 'hard-wired' with all the neurons it will need throughout life. The brain doubles in size during the first year, reaching 80 per cent of its adult volume by three years of age (Urban Child Institute 2016). The creation of synapses to connect the neurons occurs at the most prolific rate during the first three years of life when the brain generates more than twice the number it will need in adulthood. This allows the brain to construct, shape and adapt itself, according to the experiences and environmental stimuli it receives and processes during the life-course, strengthening synapses that are used repeatedly, while pruning away others that are used only rarely or not at all. The brain is a 'dynamic, ever changing biological system that is the product of our genetic potential and our history of experience' (Kapit et al. 2000). The widely held *Nature v Nurture* debate loses relevance as increasing knowledge about the interplay between genetic predisposition and lived experience offers new insight into optimal brain functioning and development (Britto 2014). This interplay can be summarized thus: 'Genes predict our brain development but it is experience that sculpts it' (ibid.).

The early stages of brain development are strongly influenced by genetic factors, with genes directing newly formed neurons to the appropriate region of the brain and determining how they will interact (Urban Child Institute 2016). The 'fine tuning' of the brain also occurs through the expression of genes, but this requires input from the environment to stimulate the neural activity. Research confirms that brain development is 'use dependent' and that the normal organization of any one region of the brain is 'dependent upon the presence, pattern, frequency and timing of experiences during development' (Perry et al. 2000: 10).

Play is an innate human trait (Rogerson et al. n.d.) and it is self-reinforcing because it makes learning fun – at the heart of all play is the pleasure drive. Pleasurable experiences activate the brain reward pathways, motivating the individual to repeat the rewarding behavior. The individual pays attention to what activates the reward pathway, forming memories which will allow for future repetition of the reward (Icahn School of Medicine 2016). In evolutionary terms, the pleasure pathway is a very old pathway which uses dopamine neurons to mediate behavior in response to both rewarding and adverse experiences (ibid.).

Individual variations in the inclination to engage in exercise as a leisure activity exemplify the interplay between neural processes and experience. The uptake of exercise as a leisure activity is believed to be a heritable characteristic linked to genes that influence the reaction to exercise in relation to the feelings of reward gained or adverse effects suffered. This has led to the suggestion that 'innate differences in dopaminergic functioning can affect physical activity behavior' (Huppertz et al. 2014). Once again, environmental factors can be shown to enhance genetic potential since exercise undertaken in natural environments, especially near water (known as blue space), is seen as being particularly beneficial to health (European Center for Environment and Human Health 2014). The brain is a social organ and exercising together with other people is an intrinsically rewarding experience (Kirkwood et al. 2008) which can encourage the uptake of exercise as a leisure activity (Cox 2012). Conversely, brain function and mental capital are adversely affected when opportunities for social engagement are absent. Loneliness – now identified as a major public health issue – has been shown to trigger genetic changes which increase the risk of premature death by up to 14 per cent (Knapton 2015). Originally associated with the older age group, loneliness is now more common among adults between 18 and 34 years of age than in those over 55, and this has been linked to an increased incidence of stroke and heart disease in this age-group (Knapton 2016). As Kirkwood et al. (2008) suggest, 'there is potential for significant gain or loss of mental capital depending on whether the reward system is appropriately stimulated' and this clearly also applies to the functionality of the brain.

Gauntlett et al. (2010) note that, aside from providing pleasure, play also stimulates perceptual, neuronal and motor development. The repetitive, consistent, and predictable elements of play help to organize and promote neural systems, which in turn develop and enhance cognitive, motor, social and emotional skills (Perry et al. 2000). Building on the work of Perry et al. (2000), Gooey Brains have summarized the significance of play as a cyclical process that is fundamental for healthy brain development:

1   A child is naturally curious.
2   The child's curiosity drives them to explore through play.
3   As the child explores through play they discover new things and learn.
4   The child finds learning and exploring fun!
5   A child likes to repeat activities that are fun.
6   Repeating fun play activities helps a child to achieve mastery of their skills.
7   A child who is mastering new skills feels confident!
8   A confident child feels capable of attempting their next challenge.

*(Gooey Brains 2015)*

Play can improve the expression of gene potential and its impact is maximized through the provision of safe, nurturing and predictable experiences (Perry et al. 2000). Sensory enrichment through a range of opportunities to see, hear, touch, taste and smell provides a global learning experience that induces associations between learning and memory (Daffner 2016). Pleasurable sensory input may inspire learning and memory, but over-stimulation of the senses may also create negative associations for some people, such as those on the autistic spectrum and those living with dementia-related conditions (Cayton 2001). Safe, nurturing and predictable experiences optimize neurobiological capabilities which in turn promote health, wellbeing, productivity and creativity for the individual, enhancing the development and reserves of mental capital. However, when these opportunities are absent or when the environment is one of neglect, fear, stress or chaos, then anxiety replaces curiosity and the drive to play is diminished or may disappear completely (Perry et al. 2000). Adverse environmental circumstances are damaging to health and wellbeing and, as demonstrated in Figure 2.1, mental capital will be wasted (Foresight Mental Capital and Wellbeing Project 2008: 3). Play and playfulness can provide a means of mitigating adverse circumstances but advocacy through the public health agenda may be necessary for play to be deployed as a force for good.

## Play, playfulness and the brain

Play and playfulness have the power to promote, protect and prolong optimal brain functioning, as well as to prevent neurological damage. Play is uniquely positioned to enable children and adults to learn through exploration and experimentation, whereby 'risk is removed, so learners can practise the skills they need to develop, without worrying about failure' (Walsh 2016). During childhood, emerging play capabilities can be mapped to the developing brain, as shown in Table 2.1, with the complexity of play behavior running parallel to the maturation of brain-related structures (Perry et al. 2000; Gooey Brains 2015).

**TABLE 2.1** Linking play to the sequential neurodevelopment of the brain.

| Stages of play (Rubin et al. 1978) | Age | Neurodevelopment sequence and functioning (Gooey Brains 2015) | Capability (Perry et al. 2000) | Play activities to encourage |
|---|---|---|---|---|
| Cooperative-constructive, socio-dynamic and games with rules | 3–6 yrs | **Neocortex** Controls concrete and abstract thoughts. As area grows, gain skills such as creativity, complex use of language, morality and respect | Encourage abstract thought humor Language Arts Games | Jokes Word games Painting/crafts Board games (Gooey Brains 2015) |
| Associative, constructive, dramatic | 1–4 yrs | **Limbic area** Emotional reactions, tolerance, empathy, affiliation. Increasingly understand social relationships | Facilitate socio-emotional growth Teams Win-Lose Turns Sharing | Simple relay games Lotto 'Simon Says' Hide and seek Skittles Teddy bear picnic |
| Parallel-functional | 6 m -2 yrs | **Midbrain** Regulates motor skills (fine and gross) Allows integration of complex sensory input | Incorporate Somato-sensory integration Large-motor skill Fine motor Music | Crawling through a tunnel Shape sorting Pots and pans Drumming (Gooey Brains 2015) |
| Solitary-functional | 0–9 m | **Brainstem** Regulates level of arousal and keeps the body functioning | Establish state regulation Peek-a-boo Taste play Tactile play | Yoghurt finger painting Sensory toys massage (Gooey Brains 2015) |

The development of play and playfulness mirrors the evolution of the brain in terms of its size and complexity. This appears to be a reciprocal arrangement since increased levels of playfulness have been linked to increasingly larger brains (Gauntlett et al. 2010). The scientific community, including 'neuroscientists, developmental biologists, psychologists, social scientists, and researchers...now know that play is a profound biological process' (Brown and Vaughan 2009) essential for optimal brain development (Gauntlett et al. 2010) and contributing to the holistic, healthy development of children and adults alike (Perry et al. 2000). This applies most notably to the frontal cortex which is responsible for higher-level cognitive functions such as monitoring behavior, divergent thinking and our ability to learn from mistakes (Gauntlett et al. 2010).

Table 2.1 links the sequence of brain development to the stages of play and suggests play activities to enhance each stage of the developmental process. It also shows how the development of humans as a playful species can be tracked from the physical play of lower order mammals through to the emergence of symbolic play in primates and the use of 'play with objects'. As the complexity of the brain evolves, 'mental representational abilities' facilitate the emergence of 'pretend play, role play, artistic expression' (Gauntlett et al. 2010: 9) in the form of music, dance, drama and the visual arts. Gray (2009) identifies activities that originate in play such as 'fun, beauty, creativity, representation [and] imagination ... as a basis for art, music, literature, theoretical science, religion and all that we call higher culture'.

Play and playfulness provide the opportunity to engage in repetitive, consistent and predictable experiences resulting in patterned neural activity that actually changes the structure of the brain (Perry et al. 2000). The positive impact of play and playfulness is not unique to the period of early development: play also facilitates the acquisition of new skills throughout the lifespan (Yeatman et al. 2014).

A great deal of research has been focused on the development of the brain during the early years, but subsequent development throughout childhood is also significant in forming attitudes and setting patterns for future health-related behavior, particularly in relation to promoting and protecting mental capital (Foresight Mental Capital and Wellbeing Project 2008). Between the ages of 10 and 12 years, increasing socialization and a move towards abstract thought allow children to think beyond their own personal experience for the first time. At this point, 'the part of the brain that regulates the processing of rewards, social feedback, and emotions becomes super sensitive' (Pevzner 2015), coinciding with a period of significant emotional, behavioral and hormonal change, which makes the young person vulnerable to risk-taking behavior (Kirkwood et al. 2008). At this stage, it is important to use 'the science of motivation and reward ... for developing new ways to secure engagement' (ibid.) which can be linked to the public health agenda and this is discussed further in Chapter 6.

## The adolescent brain

The second major phase of maturational change in the brain occurs during adolescence with the transition from 'chaos to clarity' (Willis 2016). The brain further increases in size and the prefrontal cortex reorganizes and remodels itself, resulting in the construction of the highest emotional and cognitive networks linked to executive functioning. These include organizational and planning skills, the ability to prioritize, communicate effectively, and assess risk (ibid.). The brain's potential for creativity, innovation and problem-solving continues to develop during adolescence - if the opportunities exist to practise these skills so that relevant neural networks are strengthened and reinforced (Willis 2016). Once again, play and playfulness provide the perfect means to facilitate this skill development, particularly when it comes to channelling risk-taking behavior and embracing mistakes, both of which can be powerful catalysts for learning (George Lucas Educational Foundation 2016).

At a time when pleasure is increasingly derived from social interaction with peers (Kirkwood et al. 2008), play in the form of music, drama and art can facilitate the exploration of emotions and feelings, leading to positive, enduring changes in brain biology. Many young people find the changes which accompany adolescence to be overwhelming. Figure 2.3 provides suggestions from young people themselves, of activities which can protect the brain from the risk factors associated with this crucial stage in the development of mental capital (Kirkwood et al. 2008). Many of these activities link to playful pursuits which may be associated with pleasurable childhood memories and emotions.

## The adult brain

The maturation of the brain does not stop at adolescence but is a protracted process which continues into early adulthood, particularly in the prefrontal cortex where white matter is added and synaptic pruning results in a decreasing number of connections (Rea Simpson 2008). During middle adulthood, the brain goes through a period of relative stability, adapting and changing in response to the opportunities and stresses associated with life, including work, family life and engaging with the wider society (Kirkwood et al. 2008). During adulthood, the complex interplay of factors influencing mental capital (shown in Figure 2.1) accurately reflects what happens to the adult brain. The 'wear and tear' of the normal aging process can be exacerbated by unhealthy lifestyle choices, particularly an imbalance between work and play. Playfulness is often

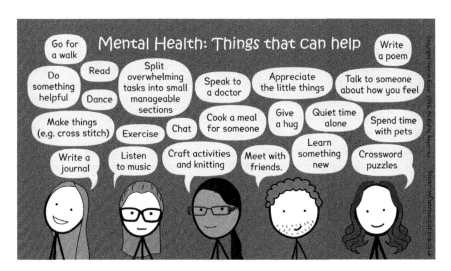

**FIGURE 2.3** Mental Health: Things that help.
Source: Ensor (2016); reproduced with kind permission of Hannah Esnor, Stickman Communications

sidelined at just the time when its restorative features and its contribution to health and wellbeing have much to offer in terms of alleviating the pressures of modern day life (Rogerson et al. n.d.; Chapter 7 addresses in more detail play's potential for improving family cohesion).

The gradual decline in mental capital mirrors the slowdown in brain processing in older age. This is thought to be due to a change in the properties of the myelin sheath that insulates electrical signals (among other things) leading to a reduction in the speed of information processing (Yeatman et al. 2014). Although brain cell degradation in old age is significant, it is not as pronounced as previously thought (Daffner 2016). In fact, neurogenesis – the growth of new neurons – particularly in the hippocampus, can enhance cognitive functioning in older age due to the brain's ability to change and adapt, in response to stimuli (ibid.). Cayton (2001) observes that 'the frailties of old age are not natural or inevitable – they are the result of systems failure', suggesting a need to embrace all efforts to promote optimal conditions for both physical and mental health in later life. The proliferation of play-based strategies for enhancing cognitive function in older age is rooted in research linked to the development of memory, which follows a similar pattern to the way in which children learn. This suggests that intergenerational activities, particularly between grandchildren and grand-parents, can be mutually beneficial for both parties and that play can provide a bridge to health across the generations.

## Play, the brain and public health

Play is particularly effective for developing and preserving procedural memory, result-ing in skills that can last a lifetime, even when other cognitive functions decline due to disease or injury (Daffner 2016). For example, patients on a hospital ward for people with dementia were often observed 'mimicking' features of their former employment such as fiddling with the springs of an upturned chair (a former mechanic) or knocking things against a wall (a former carpet fitter). Noting the creative use of their surround-ings as a means of self-stimulation through familiar activity, the design company Boex (cited in Tonkin 2016) developed a unique interactive panel which provided sensory stimulation through the application of familiar skills, for each patient on the ward.

Dolan et al. (2010) clearly identify that our behavior is heavily influenced by what grabs our attention since we unconsciously filter-out information that does not seem relevant at the time. This is a necessary coping strategy which enables us to deal with the vast amount of material processed by the brain (ibid.). However, it also means that unless health-related messages are delivered in a novel and engaging way their meaning will be lost, along with opportunities for protection and prevention. For example, a recent campaign by the Alzheimer's Society promoting brain health to teenagers in Finland (Kaijanen 2013) concluded that, while teenagers were interested in the wellbeing of their brain, they did not feel the health messages were current or relevant at their stage of life.

The Foresight Mental Capital and Wellbeing Project (2008) offers a blueprint for how we can use the predictability of brain development from conception through to early adulthood to acquire mental capital that will enhance quality of life for individuals and for society. With increasing awareness of the importance of building-up reserves of mental capital in adulthood, protecting the brain and preventing the 'systems failure' associated with injury, disease and old-age has the potential to stave off some of the diseases that have become endemic on a global level. When reserves of mental capital become depleted, the plasticity of the brain still allows for adaptation and growth, given the right conditions. Play and playfulness provide the perfect vehicle for promoting public health throughout the life-course when play is valued and encouraged for its health potential. Gauntlett et al. (2010) write:

> We find that play is at the root of many different activities that people find engaging and where communities have formed a sense of belonging and identity has also emerged, creating a compelling reason to stay engaged and return. What unifies this diverse set is less the nature of this activity, but more the 'gifts of play' that engagement in playful activities can bring.

## References

Alzheimer's Society (2014) Public Health, Prevention and Dementia, retrieved from www.alzheim ers.org.uk/site/scripts/documents_info.php?documentID=2766 (accessed 28 August 2018).

Balm, J. (2014) The Subway of the Brain – Why White Matter Matters, 14 March, retrieved from https://blogs.biomedcentral.com/on-biology/2014/03/14/the-subway-of-the-bra in-why-white-matter-matters (accessed 28 August 2018).

Britto, P. (2014) How Children's Brains Develop – New Insights, retrieved from https://blogs. unicef.org/blog/how-childrens-brains-develop-new-insights (accessed 28 August 2018).

Brown, S. (2008) Play Is More Than Just Fun, retrieved from www.ted.com/talks/stuart_ brown_says_play_is_more_than_fun_it_s_vital (accessed 28 August 2018).

Brown, S. and Vaughan, C. (2009) *Play: How it Shapes the Brain, Opens the Imagination, and Invigorates the Soul*, New York: Penguin.

Cayton, H. (2001) From Childhood to Childhood? Autonomy, Dignity and Dependence through the Ages of Life, 15th Alzheimer's Disease International Conference, Christch-urch, New Zealand, October.

Child Trauma Academy (2002) The Amazing Human Brain and Human Development: Lesson 5: Plasticity, Memory, and Cortical Modulation in the Brain, retrieved from www.childtra umaacademy.com/amazing_brain/lesson05/printing.html (accessed 28 August 2018).

Cox, S. (2012) *Game of Life: How Sport and Recreation Can Make Us Healthier, Happier and Richer, Sport and Recreation Alliance*, Sports Think Tank, retrieved from www.sportsthinkta nk.com/research,117857.html (accessed 31 December 2018).

Daffner, K. (2016) *Improving Memory: Understanding Age-Related Memory Loss*, Cambridge, MA: Harvard Medical School Patient Education Center.

Dolan, P.Hallsworth, M.Halpern, D.King, D. and Vlaev, I. (2010) *Mindspace: Influencing behaviour through Public Policy*, London: Institute for Government.

Ensor, H. (2016) 'Things that Help' Poster, retrieved from http://stickmancommunications. co.uk/epages/747384.sf/en_GB/?ObjectPath=/Shops/747384/Products/POS08/Sub Products/POS08-0001 (accessed 28 August 2018).

European Centre for Environment and Human Health (2014) Interdisciplinary Research: Blue Gym, retrieved from www.ecehh.org/research/#!blue-gym (accessed 4 December 2015).

Faculty of Public Health (2018) Concepts of Mental and Social Wellbeing, retrieved from www.fph.org.uk/policy-campaigns/special-interest-groups/special-interest-groups-list/public-mental-health-special-interest-group/better-mental-health-for-all/concepts-of-mental-and-social-wellbeing (accessed 28 August 2018).

Foresight Mental Capital and Wellbeing Project (2008) *Systems Maps: Mental Capital and Wellbeing Project*, London: The Government Office for Science.

Gauntlett, D., Ackermann, E., Whitebread, D., Wolbers, T. and Weckstrom, C. (2010) *The Future of Play. Defining the Role and Value of Play in the 21st Century*, Billund, Denmark: LEGO Learning Institute.

George Lucas Educational Foundation (2016) Learning through Mistakes, retrieved from www.edutopia.org/practice/embracing-failure-building-growth-mindset-through-arts (accessed 28 August 2018).

Gooey Brains (2015) Using Play to Build the Brain, retrieved from https://gooeybrains.com/2016/04/10/using-play-to-build-the-brain (accessed 28 August 2018).

Gray, P. (2009) Play Makes Us Human 1: A Ludic Theory of Human Nature, 4 June, retrieved from www.psychologytoday.com/blog/freedom-learn/200906/play-makes-us-human-i-ludic-theory-human-nature (accessed 28 August 2018).

Huppertz, C., Bartels, M., Groen-Blokhuis, M., Dolan, C., de Moor, M., Abdellaoui, A., van Beijsterveldt, C., Ehli, E., Hottenga, J., Willemsen, G., Xiao, X.Scheet, P., Davies, G., Boomsma, D., Hudziak, J. and de GeusE. (2014) The Dopaminergic Reward System and Leisure Time Exercise Behavior: A Candidate Allele Study, *BioMed Research International*, 2014: article 591717.

Icahn School of Medicine (2016) Brain Reward Pathways, retrieved from http://neuroscience.mssm.edu/nestler/brainRewardpathways.html (accessed 28 August 2018).

Kaijanen, S. (2013) Life Is Cool with a Fit Brain – a Brain Health Promotion Campaign for Teenagers in Alzheimer Society of Finland, retrieved from www.muistiliitto.fi/files/8313/7645/8763/Life_is_Cool_with_Fit_Brains.pdf (accessed 17 October 2016).

Kapit, W. and Elson, L. (1977) *The Anatomy Coloring Book*, New York: Harper & Row.

Kapit, W., Macey, R. and Meisami, E. (2000) *The Physiology Coloring Book*, New York: Pearson.

Kirkwood, T., Bond, J., May, C., McKeith, I. and Teh, M. (2008) *Mental Capital through Life: Future Challenges*, London: The Government Office for Science.

Knapton, S. (2015) Loneliness Triggers Biological Changes which Cause Illness and Early Death, *The Telegraph*, 23 November, retrieved from www.telegraph.co.uk/news/science/science-news/12012663/Loneliness-triggers-biological-changes-which-cause-illness-and-early-death.html (accessed 28 August 2018).

Knapton, S. (2016) Loneliness Is Public Health Problem which Raises Risk of Stroke and Heart Disease, *The Telegraph*, 19 April, retrieved from www.telegraph.co.uk/science/2016/04/19/loneliness-is-public-health-problem-which-raises-risk-of-stroke (accessed 28 August 2018).

Perry, B., Hogan, L. and Marlin, S. (2000) Curiosity, Pleasure and Play: A Neurodevelopmental Perspective, HAAEYE *Advocate*, August: 9–12.

Pevzner, H. (2015) Brain Development in Children, 10 November, retrieved from https://aldenbridgepreschool.org/blog/view/591/brain-development-in-children (accessed 28 August 2018).

Rea Simpson, A. (2008) Young Adult Development Project, retrieved from http://hrweb.mit.edu/worklife/youngadult/youngadult.pdf (accessed 28 August 2018).

Rogerson, R., Treadaway, C., Lorimer, H., Billington, J. and Fyfe, H. (n.d.) Permission to Play: Taking Play Seriously in Adulthood, retrieved from http://rjrogerson.weebly.com/

uploads/2/4/9/5/24952636/ahrc_cc_summary_report_permission_to_play.pdf   (accessed 28 August 2018).

Rubin, K.Watson, K. and Jambor, T. (1978) Free-Play Behaviors in Preschool and Kindergarten Children, *Child Development*, 49(2): 534–536.

Tonkin, A. (2016) Playful Design, in A. Tonkin, and J. Whitaker (eds), *Play in Healthcare for Adults: Using Play to Promote Health and Wellbeing Across the Adult Lifespan*, 212–225, Abingdon: Routledge.

Urban Child Institute (2016) Baby's Brain Begins Now: Conception to Age 3, retrieved from www.urbanchildinstitute.org/why-0-3/baby-and-brain (accessed 28 August 2018).

Walsh, A. (2016) Think Play Is for Nurseries, Not Universities? Think Again, retrieved from www.theguardian.com/higher-education-network/2016/sep/01/think-play-is-for-nurser ies-not-universities-think-again (accessed 28 August 2018).

Willis, J. (2016) Brain Development and Adolescent Growth Spurts, retrieved from www. edutopia.org/blog/brain-development-adolescent-growth-spurts-judy-willis (accessed 28 August 2018).

Yeatman, J., Wandell, B. and Mezer, A. (2014) Lifespan Maturation and Degeneration of Human Brain White Matter, *Nature Communications*, 5: 4932.

# 3

# THE SCIENCE OF PUBLIC HEALTH

*Alison Tonkin and Lisa Whiting*

## Introduction

In a book review by Paccaud (1999: 389), which critiques *The Potential for Health* by Kenneth Calman (former Chief Medical Officer for England), Paccaud is scathing about the significant absence of any reference to bibliographic material, suggesting that the lay public will be given 'the misleading impression that public health is much more an art than a science, a matter of opinion rather than a discipline of observation, analysis, and action'. Paccaud's disdain for the 'art' of public health epitomizes the perception that public health should be associated with scientific endeavor as the foundation of society's effort to address the biggest challenges to the health and wellbeing of the public (Academy of Medical Sciences 2018).

The Science Council (2018) defines science as 'the pursuit and application of knowledge and understanding of the natural and social world following a systematic methodology based on evidence'. Scientific enquiry covers a wide range of activities and demands exploration that is systematic and evidence-based. As such, *science* enables verification and testing of concepts, facilitating peer review and critical scrutiny of the evidence being presented (ibid.). Science provides facts and figures that result in quantifiable evidence of efficacy – proof that interventions work, and provide value for money, which is particularly useful in times of fiscal austerity. Play and playfulness come in many differing forms, which results in difficulties isolating specific and measurable outcomes of the benefits play can bestow on individuals and on society as a whole (Gordon 2014). This leaves play in a vulnerable position, meaning that play has been 'largely ignored' by most scientists studying and working in the realms of health and wellbeing (ibid.). Gordon (ibid.: 234) asserts that 'the absence of play is a serious omission', particularly when the associated benefits can be linked to the natural sciences, social sciences, neuroscience, environmental science – in fact all the scientific areas that contribute to public health.

This chapter will explore the contribution that play and playfulness can make to the scientific pursuit of public health. It will demonstrate how play and playfulness enable engagement and collaboration, promote innovation and curiosity, and advocate for protection of environments that enable play endeavors to be pursued.

## Background

Public health does not solely focus on the prevention and eradication of disease, rather, it is concerned with the whole breadth of health and wellbeing. The view that individuals are not only able to make choices about their health and wellbeing but are also able to take control of the decision-making process, has been widely accepted for many years as a central and fundamental component of health promotion (Downie et al. 1996).

Approaches to health promotion have diversified in recent years, with a broad range of options now considered; for example, Scriven et al. (2017) describe five models (Table 3.1).

Despite the diversity of approaches, success has not necessarily followed. For example, adult obesity levels continue to rise in England (Health and Social Care Information Center 2016), despite various anti-obesity campaigns. It could be argued, therefore, that it is necessary to consider how individuals, groups and communities can be helped to further engage with, and contribute to, the promotion of their own health.

Playfulness is the 'predisposition to frame (or reframe) a situation in such a way as to provide oneself (and possibly others) with amusement, humor, and/or entertainment' (Barnett 2007: 955); it is the ability of humans to be able to enjoy life (Yue et al. 2016). The need to engage and incorporate a playful and engaging approach is well established within childhood education; but it has also been suggested that play and playfulness can facilitate adult learning (Tanis 2012) and that play may have a positive

TABLE 3.1 Five models of health promotion.

| Model | Focus |
| --- | --- |
| Medical | Health is defined as the absence of disease |
| Holistic | This broadens the medical model to also incorporate the concept of positive health (in other words, the assets in people's lives that can potentially enhance their health) |
| Biopsychosocial | This also extends the medical model by including social, psychological and emotional aspects |
| Ecological | This focuses on how individuals and their environments interact with each other |
| Wellness | This has some similarities with the holistic model insomuch as it focusses on positive health and the availability of personal resources (both physical and emotional) |

Source: Scriven et al. (2017)

impact on personal perceptions of wellbeing (Proyer 2012) and happiness (Yue et al. 2016). Li et al. (2016) undertook a randomized controlled trial with 49 older adults who had a diagnosis of depression in which the participants were allocated to one of two groups to ascertain whether increased playfulness led to improvements in their depressive state. The findings indicated that this was indeed the case, with playfulness (in this case Wii Sports games) impacting positively on feelings of emotional wellbeing.

There are many opportunities to consider how public health, specifically health promotion, might further embrace a playfulness approach. For example, the need to improve physical activity levels for adults has been advocated for many years, with guidelines (Public Health England 2016) suggesting that adults (aged 19–64 years) should undertake at least 150 minutes of moderate activity each week, as well as exercise to strengthen muscles on a minimum of two days per week. While there are some excellent examples of the more traditional approaches available to adults to facilitate engagement with physical activity (such as gym, swimming and walking classes), a more playful approach has tended to focus on children's engagement. However, adults too can also benefit from more creatively playful physical activities. Paul et al. (2017) reported on Starfish, a smartphone app which was designed to increase physical activity in older adults who had survived a stroke. The app was developed to be used by groups of four people, with each person represented by a fish avatar. The fish appear in a tank on the 'wallpaper' of the smartphone and each time a person takes some steps, their fish swims into the tank and blows bubbles – and the tail and fins of the fish grow. The app is designed to keep a log of activity levels and to provide 'rewards' in the form of sea creatures who appear in the tank. The findings from the pilot study indicate that the app was not only enjoyed, but provided social support and an element of competition, as well as motivation for the users (Paul et al. 2017).

## Epidemiology

Epidemiology, which is the 'key quantitative discipline that underpins public health' (Danesh 2018), has been defined as: 'the study of the distribution and determinants of health–related states or events in specified populations, and the application of this study to the prevention and control of health problems' (Last 2001: 61).

One of the key roles of an epidemiologist is the promotion of public health via scientific enquiry and causal reasoning. Epidemiology focuses on the distribution of disease as well as the determinants of ill-health and the populations affected. For example, the World Health Organization has reported that approximately 60,000 preterm babies are born in the UK each year (World Health Organization 2012; World Health Organization 2018a), which is equivalent to 7 per cent of all live births (Office for National Statistics 2015). Further scrutiny of the data (World Health Organization 2018a) reveals that African countries have an increased incidence of premature births compared with most European countries, while the UK has a slightly higher premature birth rate (with the Black Caribbean ethnic population having the highest incidence) than a number of its European counterparts (Office for National Statistics 2015). This sort of information helps health professionals to identify the areas of health service provision that may require specific attention.

Buck-Louis et al. (2015) provide an overview of the continuing contribution epidemiology makes to public health; the authors highlight the research and development that has taken place in the key areas of cancer, nutrition, cardiovascular and infectious diseases as well as perinatal, occupational and environmental epidemiology. As stated above, a prevailing health concern in the UK is that of obesity, and epidemiologically focused research can provide an invaluable insight into the human behaviors underlying this disease. For example, Carreras-Torres et al. (2018) undertook a Mendelian randomization study using data from over 446,000 participants to ascertain whether those who have higher levels of body fat, BMI (body mass index) and waist circumference are more likely to smoke. The authors concluded that the results 'strongly suggest that higher adiposity influences smoking behavior and could have implications for the implementation of public health interventions aiming to reduce the prevalence of these important risk factors' (Carreras-Torres et al. 2018: 1). Other studies, such as that by Masi et al. (2018), have indicated that those who have increased weight gain during their mid-thirties to early forties are more likely to have lower cognitive function in later years – meaning that BMI could be an indicator of future cognitive decline.

The insight provided by epidemiology cannot be under-estimated; it has a role to play in all aspects of public health, informing health priorities at local, national and international levels. Epidemiological data is widely available (from organizations such as the Office for National Statistics, Public Health England and the World Health Organization) and it is therefore crucial that relevant information is accessed and appropriately drawn on by health professionals to underpin their practice.

## Illustrative case studies

The remaining part of this chapter will provide a more detailed exploration of a variety of current *hot topics* causing significant concern to the public health community. These will be used to demonstrate how three of the main pillars of public health activity (promotion, prevention, protection) utilize play and playfulness in synergy with scientific activity.

### Overarching public health activity – antimicrobial resistance

The pursuit of public health has historically evolved in line with the changing needs of society (Science Museum n.d.) with scientific and technological advances enabling deeper understanding of the associations between causation and subsequent action. It has been estimated that the development of antibiotic treatments has prolonged the life of every person by an average of 20 years (Longitude Prize 2018a). However, the overuse of antibiotics has simultaneously led to a global surge in anti-microbial resistance, resulting in untreatable infections which can affect any member of the global community at any time and in any place (World Health Organization 2018b).

According to the World Health Organization:

> AMR [antimicrobial resistance] is the ability of a microorganism (like bacteria, viruses, and some parasites) to stop an antimicrobial (such as antibiotics, antivirals and antimalarials) from working against it. As a result, standard treatments become ineffective, infections persist and may spread to others.
>
> *(World Health Organization 2018b)*

If action is not undertaken on a global scale, and as a matter of urgency, the potential impact has been estimated at 10 million deaths per year from 2050, at a cost of £66 trillion to the global economy due to lost productivity (Public Health England 2017a). Described as an 'antibiotic apocalypse' and the 'end of modern medicine' (Public Health England 2017b), efforts are now being made to raise awareness of the detrimental effects resulting from the overuse of antibiotics by health professionals and the public alike.

Conveying complex scientific messages in an engaging and entertaining manner means that responsibility for the health of the global community can be shared, and effective health literacy is a key tool in the public health toolkit (Dinnen and Tonkin 2016). Visualizing the pathogens that cause infections and spread disease can be a useful way of raising awareness. GIANTmicrobes manufactures over 150 different plush toy microbes that are 'a million times the actual size'. Each toy is scientifically based on an image of the microbe as seen under the microscope and can be used to open-up potentially difficult conversations in a safe and supportive manner (ibid.).

Public Health England (2017b) launched the 'Keep Antibiotics Working' campaign in 2017, in an effort to protect the public from antibiotic resistance and from a future in which antibiotics could prove ineffective at a time of need. The campaign used humor as a means of engaging the public and included advertising, the use of social media and partnership working with pharmacies. The campaign deployed engagement techniques more typically associated with marketing: a short TV advert which featured 'singing' red and white pills (Figure 3.1):

> Antibiotics – we're wonderful pills
> But don't ever think we'll cure all of your ills
> So every time you feel a bit under the weather,
> Don't always think we can make you better.
> Take us for the wrong thing – that's dangerous to do,
> When you really need us, we could stop working for you,
> So please don't end up paying the price,
> Always take your doctor's advice.
> *(Public Health England n.d; reproduced with kind permission)*

The infection control team at the Evelina Children's Hospital in London supported the 'Keep Antibiotics Working' campaign with games and information for young

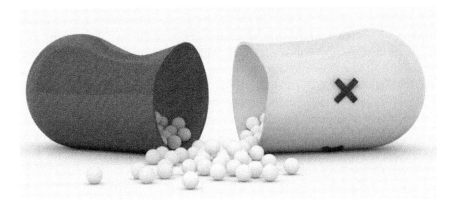

**FIGURE 3.1** 'Keep Antibiotics Working Pill'.
Source: Public Health England (2017b); reproduced with kind permission from Public Health England

people – including the appearance of a staff member dressed as a giant microbe – to raise awareness of what can be done 'by all of us' to maintain antibiotic effectiveness (Guy's and St Thomas' NHS Foundation Trust 2017). These activities coincided with World Antibiotic Awareness Week in November 2017 (World Health Organization 2018c), which has become an annual event. Campaign materials incorporated cartoon characters, including animated GIFs depicting people of differing ages and ethnicities, viruses, germs and faeces. Protection of the environment, preventing infection through good hand hygiene, and promoting the need to listen to the advice of healthcare professionals before taking antibiotics, are all featured messages, available for download from the WHO website as part of the effort to raise awareness (World Health Organization 2018d).

Playful creativity breeds novel approaches to engaging the public, and games 'can be especially effective to convey scientific content, sometimes even contributing to scientific research' (Longitude Prize 2018b). Games provide a powerful tool for engagement with complex messages (University of Plymouth 2016), enabling people to modify behavior when awareness of an important issue is raised (Gill 2017). With the advent of modern technology, games have the potential to reach a mass audience through gaming platforms, the internet and mobile devices. This potential is being embraced by game designers who, in 2016 identified antibiotic resistance as the core theme for a Games Jam Event – *Games for Better: A Games Jam on Antibiotic Resistance* (Gill 2017). Games Jams bring game developers together for a short period of time – in this instance 48 hours – to develop games from 'concept to implementation' (Gill 2017).

Although the main cause of antimicrobial resistance has been identified as the overuse of anti-microbial agents (World Health Organization 2018b), Shaw (2016) suggests that the origins of this resistance might be found in public sanitation measures designed to 'break the chain of infection'. New efforts are needed to re-engage society with simple strategies such as hand-washing, to reduce the transmission of disease (as discussed in Chapter 8), which could prevent infection in the first place (Shaw 2016). The same message was being promoted just under 100 years ago, when Winslow (1920: 26) described 'the teacher of personal hygiene … as a supremely important factor in the present-day campaign for public health'.

The National Institute for Health and Care Excellence (NICE) have published guidance advocating the importance of teaching all children and young people good hand-hygiene, and how they can independently manage some common infections (Regis and Stone 2017). NICE have endorsed a teaching tool called 'e-Bug', an educational software package featuring interactive games for children which are differentiated according to age/stage and developmental level (Regis and Stone 2017). Developed by Public Health England, e-Bug features a range of games designed to teach the core messages around effective personal hygiene, useful and harmful microbes, and the importance of finishing a course of antibiotics. There is also a six-week community course for those delivering the e-Bug programme within community groups and settings called 'Beat the Bugs Train the Trainer', which promotes *fun* as a key component of each training session (e-Bug, 2017).

## *Promotion – salutogenesis*

Antonovsky (1979) coined the term 'salutogenesis', derived from the Latin *salus* meaning health, safety, and wellbeing, and the Greek work *genesis* meaning origin – in other words the 'origins of health' (Antonovsky 1996: 13). Antonovsky (ibid.: 11) thought of salutogenesis as a 'more viable paradigm for health promotion research and practice' than the 'disease orientation' model since it focuses on 'moving people in the direction of the health end of a healthy/dis-ease continuum'. Antonovsky (ibid.) believed that there existed the potential to enhance the health of *all* people, irrespective of their current health status, suggesting that the focus of health promotion should be on the whole person rather than on their specific disease (or their risk of acquiring an illness). Antonovsky (1987: 13) commented that if he had to identify the most important aspect of salutogenesis, he would say that it 'not only opens the way for, but compels us to devote our energies to, the formulation and advance of a theory of coping'.

Antonovsky (1996) suggested that the resources exist to help people cope with stressful situations, referring to these as general resistance resources (GRRs). GRRs cover a range of biological, material (such as money) and psychosocial factors, which were identified in Antonovsky's previous independent research and peer collaborations – notably, a study that investigated how women from different cultures coped with the stress of the menopause (Datan et al. 1981).

The identification of the GRRs led Antonovsky (1987) to propose the concept of 'Sense Of Coherence' (SOC) which offers a view of the world as 'comprehensible', 'manageable' and 'meaningful' (Antonovsky 1996: 15) as shown in Table 3.2. Antonovsky (1987) suggested that an SOC is a major determinant of one's position on the

**TABLE 3.2** Central components of a sense of coherence.

| Component | Description |
|---|---|
| Comprehensibility | The extent to which sense/order can be drawn from the situation, ability to process both familiar and unfamiliar stimuli. |
| Manageability | Resources may be multi-faceted and include friends, family, God and colleagues. |
| Meaningfulness | If a person with a high degree of meaningfulness faces a difficulty, they may not be happy about it, but they are willing to face the challenge. In practical terms, the person with a strong sense of coherence will: <br>• believe that the challenge is understood (comprehensibility);<br>• believe that the resources to cope are available (manageability);<br>• be motivated to cope (meaningfulness). |

Source: Antonovsky (1987); Antonovsky (1996)

health/dis-ease continuum and of one's progression towards health. A strong SOC enables a person to respond flexibly to demands, and develops throughout childhood, adolescence and adulthood (ibid.). An individual's SOC is dependent on a range of factors including developmental stage, social circumstances, socialization within the family, gender, genetics, ethnicity and chance (Antonovsky 1996). This supports the view that it is important to create an environment in which children and young people experience consistency and within which they can recover from stress with appropriate support and have opportunities to participate in decision-making processes.

The value of a salutogenic approach to health has been demonstrated in the research (García-Moya and Morgan 2016; McCuaig and Quennerstedt 2018). There has been a recognition of the value of a salutogenic perspective in terms of the importance of outdoor space in healthcare settings (Bengtsson and Grahn 2014), while other authors (such as Buck et al. 2015; Koohsari et al. 2015) have alluded to the salutogenic effect of undertaking physical activity in green space.

Miller et al. (2014) reported on the Scottish Government's GreenHealth project which used a wide range of data collection methods to examine the relationship between green space and health in urban areas of Scotland. The findings revealed that the availability of green space and open areas positively influenced health and wellbeing; promoted physical activity, mental and social health; and reduced health inequalities. Miller et al. (ibid.) provided specific examples of the use of green space which highlight the importance of playfulness and enjoyment:

• For children, green space was a place to play with friends and an area where they were able to take advantage of the natural environment (the trees, bushes, fishing in the burn).
• The peace-and-quiet associated with green space was appreciated by both adults and children. It was an ideal environment in which to meet friends, to enjoy physical exercise, and to walk the dog.

Miller et al. (2014: 33) suggest that the 'results mark a step forward in our understanding of possible mechanisms behind any salutogenic green space effect'. The salutogenic approach can be aligned with playfulness in other areas of health; by maximizing general resistance resources (such as friends, family, pets, support organizations) people can be encouraged to enjoy activities across a range of circumstances on the health-illness continuum – the elderly lady with dementia can, for example, spend time enjoying bingo at a lunch club, thus lessening feelings of social isolation and promoting a more positive quality of life.

## Prevention – bullying

The UK government (UK Government 2018) has stated that, in terms of the law, there is no definition of bullying; however, they assert that bullying typically includes behavior that is:

- recurrent;
- intentional; and
- frequently aimed at subsectors of society (for example, related to faith, culture or sexual orientation).

Bullying is usually categorized into four groups: verbal, physical, relational and cyber, and the NSPCC (2018) suggest that it can include a wide range of activities:

- verbal language;
- non-verbal messages (could be via text or using inappropriate hand/finger signals);
- behavior that could be perceived as threatening or intimidating;
- excluding someone from activities or socially isolating them;
- trying to control someone;
- continually criticizing someone;
- bullying that is racial, sexual or homophobic;
- physical activities towards someone;
- online activities; and
- anonymous or hoax phone calls (NSPCC 2018).

Traditionally, bullying has been associated with school-aged children and young people, with several studies focusing on this age-group (for example, Chester et al. 2015; Chester et al. 2017). However, it is now recognized that bullying affects a wide range of people, with research highlighting bullying in British hospitals (Carter et al. 2013) as well as in the wider workplace (Rodríguez-Muñoz et al. 2010).

There is evidence to suggest that bullying can have long-term negative consequences which can impact on the health and wellbeing of those affected – both victims and perpetrators (Quinn and Stewart 2018). It has been suggested that bullying can result in physical symptoms, such as headaches (Due et al. 2005), bed-wetting and stomach-aches (Fekkes et al. 2006), as well as mental health problems such as depression (Bowes et al. 2015). Bullying has also been linked to unhealthy behaviors such as smoking (Vieno et al. 2011) and alcohol and drug use (Quinn and Stewart 2018). Hence, bullying has become a matter of public health concern (Anthony et al. 2010).

Health protection aims to make it easier for people to make healthy choices, but it also recognizes the socio-economic factors that can influence the promotion of health. One of the central goals of health protection is to enhance empowerment so that people feel they are in control of their lives and can make appropriate decisions (Whiting and Miller 2005). Increased awareness of the actual and potential health problems associated with bullying has led to a range of strategies to both reduce the incidence of bullying and to assist with the reporting of it – protecting those at risk and preventing its manifestation. For example, the UK Government (2016) raised awareness of an app that was supported by Government funding. Tootoot (2018) is a platform that facilitates the reporting of bullying by children and young people, via the use of screenshots of social media, and provides twenty-four-hour support for victims. Resources such as *The Anti-Bullying Game* (Steng 1996) have been designed specifically for children and young people to aid their understanding of some of the factors that underpin bullying behavior and to facilitate discussion within a 'safe' group.

It has been suggested that more creative strategies could be helpful in terms of detecting bullying. Álvarez-Bermejo et al. (2016), following initial data collection, designed a mobile phone app that involved both students and teachers. The app (PREVER: Prevention of Racial Stigma) was designed for young people under the age of 16 years and specifically focused on the identification of racially based bullying through gamification. When a student interacted with the app, s/he was both player and subject of the game. This afforded the player the experience of reflecting on their actions towards others, both as victim and as perpetrator in a racial bullying scenario.

Many anti-bullying initiatives have focused on more traditional education approaches: for example, school-based student and teacher training programmes, peer-to-peer anti-bullying ambassadors and helplines – all of which are to be applauded for their positive contribution to the anti-bullying agenda. However, creative approaches such as the PREVER app could augment such mainstream strategies by offering alternative methods of engagement which are both protective and empowering, and which facilitate self-reflection, as well as having the potential to identify inappropriate discriminatory and/or bullying behaviors.

## Protection – topophilia

The National Trust is a conservation charity independent of the UK Government which, more than 120 years after it was founded, cares for over 600,000 acres of countryside, 775 miles of coastline and hundreds of special places across England, Wales and Northern Ireland (National Trust 2017: 43). A few years prior to the founding of the National Trust in 1895, the co-founder Olivia Hill described the founding principles of the National Trust, namely:

'We all need space; unless we have it we cannot reach that sense of quiet in which whispers of better things come to us gently... places to sit in, places to play in, places to stroll in, and places to spend a day in' (National Trust 2017: 27). Hill (cited in National Trust 2017: 3) went on to describe '...the need for quiet, the need for air, and I believe the sight of sky and of things growing, [which] seem human needs, common to all'. The National Trust (ibid.) propose that the human need to engage with the natural world illustrates the concept of topophilia (Greek *topos* – 'place' – and *philia* – 'love of') which describes the 'visceral but intangible feeling' of the attachment we have to places.

There is significant qualitative evidence that supports the need for humans to engage with nature and the natural world, as shown in Figure 3.2.

Marmot (2010: 24) recommended that access to, and improvement of, the availability of 'good quality open and green spaces across the social gradient' should be integrated into policy to reduce health inequalities.

However, scientific evidence is still considered to be the 'gold standard' when it comes to defining efficacy (Science Council 2018). This point is echoed by the National Trust (2018) who state 'we've always believed that natural and historic places have a powerful effect on all of us. Now, for the first time, there's scientific proof'. With the advent of new imaging technologies such as functional Magnetic Resonance

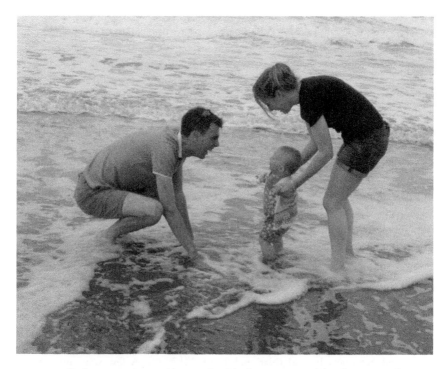

**FIGURE 3.2** Early connections with meaningful places protected by the National Trust. Source: photograph of Jenni, Kevin and Grace Etchells by Alison Tonkin

Imaging (fMRI) scientific evidence to support tacit knowledge is more widely available, and the National Trust (NT) used fMRI evidence as part of a major research project titled Places That Make Us (National Trust 2017). Using a triangulation approach, the research consisted of three strands:

- fMRI scans of 20 volunteers visualizing areas of the brain associated with processing emotional responses;
- qualitative in-depth interviews with 11 members of the public (members and non-members of the National Trust); and
- a quantitative survey with over 2000 respondents

One of the most important findings was that images can elicit strong emotional responses to places which have personal meaning to people. For those who are no longer able to visit their meaningful place, images can be used to generate feelings of connection, peace and belonging, all of which contribute to the protective mechanisms associated with emotional and mental wellbeing (National Trust 2017). The research was undertaken to demonstrate the importance of the work undertaken by the National Trust (ibid.: 43) to protect and preserve our national heritage. With over 5 million members, 620,000 volunteers and 22 million visitors each year, the National Trust has presented a scientific research base which can be used as a powerful means of advocacy if government policy should threaten access to, and enjoyment of, urban or rural places that hold meaning to people and their significant others.

## Conclusion

Public health is dependent on the wide-ranging forms and functions of scientific endeavor for securing health and wellbeing for every member of society at individual, local, national and international levels. Scientific enquiry has historically relied on the integration of quantifiable evidence arising from systematic, methodologically defined exploration. This has meant that the contribution of play and playfulness, which often fall beyond the parameters of measurable outcomes, has largely been ignored by the scientific community. However, with the advent of new technologies, and an appreciation of how play-based strategies can be used as a means of facilitating participation and engagement with the public health agenda, play and playfulness have an important contribution to make to the science of public health. This is noted by Brown (2008), who simply states: *Science + Play = Transformation.*

## References

Academy of Medical Sciences (2018) About, retrieved from https://acmedsci.ac.uk/about (accessed 11 June 2018).
Álvarez-Bermejo, J., Belmonte-Ureña, L., Martos-Martínez, A., Barragán-Martín, A. and Del Mar Simón-Marquez. M (2016) System to Detect Racial-Based Bullying through Gamification, *Frontiers in Psychology*, 7(1791): 1–13.

Anthony, B., Wessler, S. and Sebian, J. (2010) Commentary: Guiding A Public Health Approach to Bullying, *Journal of Pediatric Psychology*, 35(10): 1113–1115.

Antonovsky, A. (1979) *Health, Stress and Coping*, San Francisco, CA: Josey-Bass.

Antonovsky, A. (1987) *Unravelling the Mystery of Health: How People Manage Stress and Stay Well*, San Francisco, CA: Josey-Bass.

Antonovsky, A. (1996) The Salutogenic Model as a Theory to Guide Health Promotion, *Health Promotion International*, 11(1): 11–18.

Barnett, L. A. (2007) The Nature of Playfulness in Young Adults, *Personality and Individual Differences*, 43(4): 949–958.

Bengtsson, A. and Grahn, P. (2014) Outdoor Environments in Healthcare Settings: A Quality Evaluation Tool for Use in Designing Healthcare Gardens, *Urban Forestry and Urban Greening*, 13(4): 878–891.

Bowes, L., Joinson, C., Wolke, D., and Lewis, G. (2015) Peer Victimisation during Adolescence and its Impact on Depression in Early Adulthood: Prospective Cohort Study in the United Kingdom, *BMJ (Clinical Research Edition)*, 350: h2469.

Brown, S. (2008) Play Is More Than Just Fun, retrieved from www.ted.com/talks/stuart_brown_says_play_is_more_than_fun_it_s_vital (accessed 17 Ocotber 2016).

Buck, C., Tkaczick, T., Pitsiladis, Y., De Bourdehaudhuij, I., Reisch, L., Ahrens, W. and Pigeot, I. (2015) Objective Measures of the Built Environment and Physical Activity in Children: from Walkability to Moveability, *Journal of Urban Health*, 92(1): 24–38.

Buck-Louis, G., Bloom, M. , Gatto, N., Hogue, C., Westreich, D. and Zhang, C. (2015) Epidemiology's Continuing Contribution to Public Health: The Power of 'Then and Now', *American Journal of Epidemiology*, 181(8): e1–8.

Carter, M., Thompson, N., Crampton, P., Morrow, G., Burford, B., Gray, C. and Illing, J. (2013) Workplace Bullying in the UK NHS: A Questionnaire and Interview Study on Prevalence, Impact and Barriers to Reporting, *BMJ Open*, 3(6): e002628.

Carreras-Torres, R., Johansson, M., Haycock, P. C., Relton, C. L., Davey Smith, G., Brennan, P. and Martin, R. M. (2018) Role of Obesity in Smoking behaviour: Mendelian Randomisation Study in UK Biobank, *BMJ*, 361: k1767.

Chester, K., Callaghan, M., Cosma, A., Donnelly, P., Craig, W., Walsh, S., and Molcho, M. (2015) Cross-National Time Trends in Bullying Victimization in 33 Countries among Children Aged 11, 13 and 15 from 2002 to 2010, *The European Journal of Public Health*, 25 (suppl 2): 61–64.

Chester, K., Spencer, N., Whiting, L. and Brooks, F. (2017) Association Between Experiencing Relational Bullying and Adolescent Health-Related Quality of Life, *Journal of School Health*, 87(11): 865–872.

Danesh, J. (2018) Epidemiology and Public Health, retrieved from www.medschl.cam.ac.uk/research/research-themes/epidemiology-and-public-health (accessed 11 June 2018).

Datan, N., Antonovsky, A. and Maoz, B. (1981) *A Time to Reap: The Middle Age of Women in Five Israeli Subcultures*, Baltimore, MD: John Hopkins University Press.

Dinnen, S. and Tonkin, A. (2016) Playing with Words, in A. Tonkin, and J. Whitaker (eds), *Play in Healthcare for Adults: Using Play to Promote Health and Wellbeing Across the Adult Lifespan*, 160–172, Abingdon: Routledge.

Downie, R. S., Tannahill, C. and Tannahill, A. (1996) *Health Promotion: Models and Values*, 2nd edition, Oxford: Oxford University Press.

Due, P., Holstein, B., Lynch, J., Diderichsen, F., Gabhain, S., Scheidt, P. and Currie, C. (2005) Bullying and Symptoms among School-Aged Children: International Comparative Cross Sectional Study in 28 Countries, *European Journal of Public Health*, 15(2): 128–132.

e-Bug (2017) Online: e-Bug Training Module for Educators, retrieved from www.e-bug.eu/training.aspx?cc=eng&ss=1&t=Training (accessed 26 January 2018).

Fekkes, M., Pijpers, F., Fredriks, A., Vogels, T. and Verloove-Vanhorick, S. (2006) Do Bullied Children Get Ill, or Do Ill Children Get Bullied? A Prospective Cohort Study on the Relationship between Bullying and Health-Related Symptoms, *Pediatrics*, 117(5): 1568–1574.

García-Moya, I. and Morgan, A. (2016) The Utility of Salutogenesis for Guiding Health Promotion: The Case for Young People's Well-being, *Health Promotion International*, 32 (4): 723–733.

Gill, J. (2017) Games for Better: A Game Jam on Antibiotic Resistance, retrieved from https://longitudeprize.org/blog-post/games-better-game-jam-antibiotic-resistance (accessed 26 January 2018).

Gordon, G. (2014) Well Played: The Origins and Future of Playfulness, *American Journal of Play*, 6(2): 234–266.

Guy's and St Thomas' NHS Foundation Trust (2017) Will You Help to Keep Antibiotics Working?, retrieved from www.guysandstthomas.nhs.uk/news-and-events/2017-news/november/20171121-will-you-help-to-keep-antibiotics-working.aspx (accessed 25 January 2018).

Health and Social Care Information Centre (2016) Statistics on Obesity, Physical Activity and Diet. England 2016, retrieved from https://digital.nhs.uk/catalogue/PUB20562 (accessed 5 January 2018).

Koohsari, M.J., Mavoa, S., Villianueva, K., Sugiyama, T., Badland, H., Kaczynski, A., Owen, N. and Giles-Corti, B. (2015) Public Open Space, Physical Activity, Urban Design and Public Health: Concepts, Methods and Research Agenda, *Health and Place*, 33 (2015): 75–82.

Last, J. M. (2001) (Ed) *Dictionary of Epidemiology*, 4th edition, New York: Oxford University Press.

Li, J., Theng, Y. and Foo, S. (2016) Exergames for Older Adults with Subthreshold Depression: Does Higher Playfulness Lead to Better Improvement in Depression?, *Journal of Games Health*, 5(3): 175–182.

Longitude Prize (2018a) The Challenge: Reduce the Use of Antibiotics, retrieved from https://longitudeprize.org/challenge (accessed 27 January 2018).

Longitude Prize (2018b) Superbugs: The Game, retrieved from https://longitudeprize.org/superbugs (accessed 27 January 2018).

McCuaig, L. and Quennerstedt, M. (2018) Health by Stealth – Exploring the Sociocultural Dimensions of Salutogenesis for Sport, Health and Physical Education Research, *Sport, Education and Society*, 23(2): 111–122.

Marmot, M. (2010) *Fair Society Healthy Lives* (Full Report), London: The Marmot Review.

Masi, S., Georgiopoulos, G., Khan, T., Johnson, W., Wong, A., Charakida, M., Whincup, P., Hughes, A. D., Richards, M., Hardy, R. and Deanfield, J. (2018) Patterns of Adiposity, Vascular Phenotypes and Cognitive Function in the 1946 British Birth Cohort, *BMC Medicine*, 16(75): 1–12.

Miller, D., Morrice, J., Aspinall, P., Brewer, M., Brown, K., Cummins, R., Dilley, R., Dinnie, L., Donaldson-Selby, G., Gilbert, A., Hester, A., Harthill, P., Mitchell, R., Morris, S., Pearce, I., Robertson, L., Roe, J., Ward Thompson, C. and Wang, C. (2014) *Contribution of Green and Open Space to Public Health and Wellbeing*, Project No. MLU/ECA/UGW/847/08, Final Report, for Rural and Environmental Science and Analytical Services Division, Scottish Government, retrieved from www.hutton.ac.uk/sites/default/files/files/projects/GreenHealth-Final-Report.pdf (accessed 27 February 2018).

National Trust (2017) *Places That Make Us: Research Report*, Swindon: National Trust.

National Trust (2018) Why Do Places Mean So Much?, retrieved from www.nationaltrust.org.uk/stories/why-do-places-mean-so-much (accessed 14 April 2018).

NSPCC (2018) What are Bullying and Cyberbullying, retrieved from www.nspcc.org.uk/p reventing-abuse/child-abuse-and-neglect/bullying-and-cyberbullying/what-is-bullying-cyberbullying (accessed 24 May 2018).

Office for National Statistics (2015) Pregnancy and Ethnic Factors Influencing Births and Infant Mortality: 2013. Death Rates of Pre-Term, Full-Term and Post-Term Babies and Various Factors that May Influence Their Survival, retrieved from www.ons.gov.uk/peop lepopulationandcommunity/healthandsocialcare/causesofdeath/bulletins/pregnancyandeth nicfactorsinfluencingbirthsandinfantmortality/2015-10-14 (accessed 30 May 2018).

Paccaud, F. (1999) Book Review: The Potential for Health, *BMJ*, 319(7206): 389.

Paul, L., Brewster, S., Wyke, S., McFadyen, Sattar, N., Gill, J., Dybus, A. and Gray, C. (2017) Increasing Physical Activity in Older Adults Using Starfish, an Interactive Smart-phone Application (App); A Pilot Study, *Journal of Rehabilitation and Assistive Technologies Engineering*, 4: 1–10.

Proyer, R. (2012) Examining Playfulness in Adults: Testing its Correlates with Personality, Positive Psychological Functioning, Goal Aspirations, and Multi-methodically Assessed Ingenuity, *Psychological Test and Assessment Modeling*, 54(2): 103–127

Public Health England (2016) Health Matters: Getting Every Adult Active Every Day, retrieved from www.gov.uk/government/publications/health-matters-getting-every-adult-active-e very-day/health-matters-getting-every-adult-active-every-day (accessed 5 January 2018).

Public Health England (2017a) Health Matters: Preventing Infections and Reducing Anti-microbial Resistance, retrieved from www.gov.uk/government/publications/health-ma tters-preventing-infections-and-reducing-amr/health-matters-preventing-infections-a nd-reducing-antimicrobial-resistance (accessed 25 January 2018).

Public Health England (2017b) Taking Antibiotics When You Don't Need Them Puts You at Risk, retrieved from www.gov.uk/government/news/taking-antibiotics-when-you-dont-need-them-puts-you-at-risk (accessed 25 January 2018).

Public Health England (2018) About Us, retrieved from www.gov.uk/government/organisa tions/public-health-england/about (accessed 25 January 2018).

Public Health England (n.d.) Keep Antibiotics Working: National TV Advertisement, retrieved from https://campaignresources.phe.gov.uk/resources/campaigns/58-keep-anti biotics-working/resources/2493 (accessed 26 January 2018).

Quinn, S. and Stewart, M. (2018) Examining the Long-Term Consequences of Bullying on Adult Substance Use, *American Journal of Criminal Justice*, 43(1): 85–101.

Regis, T. and Stone, J. (2017) Children and Young People Should Be Taught Simple Hygiene Measures to Help Curb the Spread of Infections, retrieved from http://indepth. nice.org.uk/children-and-young-people-should-be-taught-simple-hygiene-measur es-to-curb-the-spread-of-infections-says-nice/index.html (accessed 26 January 2018).

Rodríguez-Muñoz, A., Moreno-Jiménez, B., Isabel Sanz Vergel, A. and Garrosa Hernández, E. (2010) Post-Traumatic Symptoms among Victims of Workplace Bullying: Exploring Gender Differences and Shattered Assumptions, *Journal of Applied Social Psychology*, 40(10): 2616–2635.

Science Council (2018) Our Definition of Science, retrieved from https://sciencecouncil. org/about-science/our-definition-of-science (accessed 13 April 2018).

Science Museum (n.d.) Public Health, retrieved from www.sciencemuseum.org.uk/brought tolife/themes/publichealth (accessed 23 June 2017).

Scriven, A., Ewles, L. and Simnett, I. (2017) *Ewles & Simnett's Promoting Health: A Practical Guide*, 7th edition, Edinburgh: Elsevier.

Shaw, K. (2016) Beating E. *Coli* – What Are You Doing to Break the Chain of Infection?, retrieved from https://publichealthmatters.blog.gov.uk/2016/10/16/beating-e-coli-wha t-are-you-doing-to-break-the-chain-of-infection (accessed 25 January 2018).

Steng, I. (1996) *The Anti-Bullying Game*, London: Jessica Kingsley Publishers.

Tanis, D. (2012) Exploring Play/Playfulness and Learning in the Adult and Higher Education Classroom, dissertation, retrieved from https://etda.libraries.psu.edu/catalog/16086 (accessed 5 January 2018).

Tootoot (2018) Giving a Voice: To Children and Young People, retrieved from https://tootoot.co.uk (accessed 11 June 2018).

UK Government (2016) Thousands More Children to Benefit from Anti-bullying App, retrieved from www.gov.uk/government/news/thousands-more-children-to-benefit-from-anti-bullying-app (accessed 24 May 2018).

UK Government (2018) Bullying at School, retrieved from www.gov.uk/bullying-at-school (accessed 24 May 2018).

University of Plymouth (2017) Games for Better: 48 Hour Game Jam for Antibiotic Resistance Awareness, retrieved from www.plymouth.ac.uk/whats-on/games-for-better (accessed 26 January 2018).

Vieno, A., Gini, G. and Santinello, M. (2011) Different Forms of Bullying and Their Association to Smoking and Drinking Behavior in Italian Adolescents, *Journal of School Health*, 81(7): 393–399.

Whiting, L. and Miller, S. (2005) Health Promotion in Community Children's Nursing, in A. Sidey and D. Widdas (eds), *Textbook of Community Children's Nursing*, 2nd edition, 149–160, London: Elsevier.

Winslow, C. (1920) The Untilled Fields of Public Health, *Science*, 51(1306): 23–33.

World Health Organization (2012) Country Data and Rankings for Preterm Birth, retrieved from www.who.int/pmnch/media/news/2012/201204_borntoosoon_countryranking.pdf (accessed 30 May 2018).

World Health Organization (2018a) Preterm Birth, retrieved from www.who.int/newsroom/fact-sheets/detail/preterm-birth (accessed 30 May 2018).

World Health Organization (2018b) Antimicrobial Resistance, retrieved from www.who.int/antimicrobial-resistance/en (accessed 25 January 2018).

World Health Organization (2018c) World Antibiotic Awareness Week, 13–19 November 2017, retrieved from www.who.int/campaigns/world-antibiotic-awareness-week/en (accessed 25 January 2018).

World Health Organization (2018d) World Antibiotics Week: Animated GIFs, retrieved from www.who.int/campaigns/world-antibiotic-awareness-week/2017/social-media/en (accessed 26 January 2018).

Yue, X., Leung, C.-L. and Hiranandani, N. (2016) Adult Playfulness, Humor Styles, and Subjective Happiness, *Psychological Reports*, 119(3): 630–640.

# 4

# THE ART OF PUBLIC HEALTH AND THE WISDOM OF PLAY

## Participation in the creative arts as a route to health and wellbeing

*Eric Fleming and Julia Whitaker*

## Introduction

A concern for good health is a recurring refrain for most people, and one with which we become familiar during our formative years (OECD n.d.). However, the 'healthy living' mantra, communicated by parents, educators, health professionals and government policy, risks becoming so embedded in the cultural environment that its meaning and impact diminish with frequent repetition (Womack 2005). For most people, risk-taking and the drive for wellness are held in balance (Cook and Bellis 2001) such that life becomes fruitful in terms of educational achievement, family life, career development and the potential for autonomy and self-esteem. 'Healthy living' has come to mean more than simply how we feel in our physical bodies; the term also implies that we have the developmental opportunities to discover the different aspects of ourselves, to realize personal potential, and to form healthy attachments to others and to place. This is supported by research carried out at the Stanford Prevention Research Center which found that the ten most commonly cited dimensions of wellness were 'social connectedness, lifestyle behaviors, stress and resilience, emotional health, physical health, meaning and purpose, sense of self, finances, spirituality or religiosity, and exploration and creativity' (Heaney 2017).

Adults with learning disabilities encounter more limited opportunities to contribute to the drawing of a personal life-map by which they might discover or realize this deeper, more personal sense of wellness and the associated self-esteem (Independent Living Strategy Group 2015). They also commonly experience a range of secondary health issues (Public Health England 2018) and may carry a history of psychological trauma (Wigham and Emerson 2015). There is now an established body of evidence (APPG on Arts, Health and Wellbeing 2017) to show that, when people are suffering, either physically or emotionally, and are at a low-ebb in terms of self-esteem, the playful, creative self-expression found in art, drama, dance and music, can help to restore emotional balance (e.g. Jenson 2013) and to renew a focus on health-giving activity (Impact Arts 2011).

This chapter examines the role of playful involvement in the creative arts in relation to the creation of a healthy community (Stuckey and Nobel 2010). It uses a case-study approach to describe and discuss aspects of play in participatory art, in the context of a project planned and delivered by members of the glass studio at Garvald Edinburgh, an organization offering support and creative opportunities to adults with learning disabilities (see www.garvaldedinburgh.org.uk).

## Health, autonomy and self-esteem

Sennett (2003) argues that we live in a society of pervasive inequalities – inequalities in natural ability, in life chances, and in achievement – and that these inequalities are reflected in disparities in respect and in self-esteem. Self-esteem is closely linked with autonomy and the availability of opportunities to achieve self-respect. Doyal and Gough (1991) hold that health and autonomy are the only two basic human needs and Marmot (2003) expands on this, stating: 'Individuals do not worry about the means of achieving good health and only then concern themselves with autonomy … Low levels of autonomy and low self-esteem are likely to be related to worse health' (Marmot 2003: 574). Inequalities experienced at the start of life have a continuing effect throughout the lifespan and our 'position on the social gradient' is a determining factor in terms of health and wellbeing (APPG on Arts, Health and Wellbeing 2017: 118). While health equity remains a public health priority, attention must be given to equitable opportunities for achieving autonomy and self-esteem (Deci and Ryan 1995) and engagement in the arts has been found to play a central role in overturning predestined outcomes (APPG on Arts, Health and Wellbeing 2017: 118).

Therapeutic arts-and-crafts, and the play and playfulness experienced through such activities, can free the energies of expression, choice, and aspiration which underlie a sense of autonomy and of self (Burt and Atkinson 2011). This selfhood is then reflected in community recognition and appreciation, reinforcing in the individual a sense of having a unique contribution to make to their community (Public Broadcasting Service 2018). Without such an outlet, the need and aspiration to actively engage with the community may lay dormant and frustrated, resulting in social isolation and low self-esteem (Wilson et al. 2017). Low self-esteem can 'lead to health damaging behaviors and to activation of biological stress mechanisms that increase risk of diseases such as coronary heart disease' (Marmot 2003).

## Rudolf Steiner and creative endeavor as a route to wellness

Garvald Edinburgh is an organization inspired by the philosophy of Rudolf Steiner, a philosophy which he termed '*anthroposophy*', meaning 'awareness of one's humanity' (James 2001: 239). This formal educational, therapeutic, and creative system seeks to use mainly natural means to optimize physical, mental and spiritual health and wellbeing (Dictionary.com 2018). Steiner postulated that craft-based practice provides a sense of purpose, of belonging, and of achievement which contributes to both the physical health and the emotional wellbeing of adults with learning disabilities. This can be understood in terms of the impact of practical activities on the 'internal locus of control'. Sigman (2015) explains: 'It seems that by learning to control things in a "hands-on" context, students gain a more general sense of control over other areas of their lives'. Opportunities to actively engage in the process of creative arts-and-crafts as part of a micro-community can prove helpful to individuals with additional support needs because they provide a foot-hold on life's journey – today experienced as an increasingly more complex and unpredictable task, given the fragmentation of service-provision and uncertain funding (Mencap 2012).

Among his many initiatives, Steiner developed unique approaches to the edu-cation and care of children and of adults with learning disabilities, which he termed *curative education* and *social therapy* (Curative Education and Social Therapy Council 2018). The practice of arts-and-crafts was promoted as an opportunity for practical, artistic and social development, which would enable participants to find balance in 'thinking, feeling and willing', thus realizing their potential to live meaningful lives (ibid.). The creative, consistent, and rhythmical pace of the supported skill acquisition inherent to arts-and-crafts practice is at the core of this balance. The key aspects of skill acquisition in any craft are not easily negotiated in isolation, but are learnt through observation, trial-and-error, and with the support of experienced practitioners who are willing and able to share their knowledge and skills (Sennett 2008). Steiner suggested that practitioners in this supportive role should 'become like dancers' and be 'versatile in their approach and attitude' to meeting the needs of others (Garvald Edinburgh 2003: 3).

The designation 'social' therapy implies that the relational aspects of community and society are central to its aims (Curative Education and Social Therapy Council 2018). A social therapy model recognizes the pendulum swing of correspondence between the individual and the community as the stage-setting for life-learning. The individual both influences and is influenced by their social environment, according to the principles of reciprocal determinism (Bandura 1978). The self-image which is expressed in a social context, and then reflected by the community, is intimately related to a sense of self-respect and of self-esteem.

A concern for the relational aspect is something which social therapy shares with *relational aesthetics*, a term coined by Bourriard in the 1990s 'to describe the tendency to make art based on, or inspired by, human relations and their social context' (Tate 2018). The historical transition from art as object to art as experience shifted the relationship between people and the significant art object such that it 'is now focused on inter-human relations' which have 'become fully fledged artistic forms' (Bourriaud 2002: 28). Bourriaud's description of the relational, matches the aims of an organization such as Garvald Edinburgh whose social therapy ethos is similarly intended to foster meaningful encounter (Garvald Edinburgh 2003).

## Play as an agent of creative engagement

In the glass studio, one of several craft workshops run by Garvald Edinburgh, the expression of play is evident in various forms. Play is manifest throughout the creative process in imaginative experimentation with shape, color, form and material. Playful banter and humor punctuate purposeful dialogue and conversation. A natural, spontaneous sense of play, when allowed to flow freely between people, is like light streaming into a previously darkened room: it has an energy which can ignite positivity and open-up relational bonds through the experience of feeling acknowledged, appreciated and recognized. This playful energy is the starting-point from which people can more easily engage with creative activities, finding self-expression through color and form. A playful approach reduces inhibitions and awakens the potential for free expression in a mode best suited to the individual. Creating and doing are intuitive processes which allow the imagination 'more room to play' (Tite et al. 2016: 28), and the qualitative nature of arts-and-crafts activities represents a visual language which is animated through this playful experimentation (Warburton 2017).

In an organization which provides creative and therapeutic activities for adults with learning disabilities, engagement with play can be helpful in bringing people together; in animating a social space; and in motivating creative energy and practice. Play is cultivated for both its therapeutic and its expressive potential, transforming the studio space into a fertile ground for witnessing how play can contribute to health and wellbeing through its influence on a sense of purpose and self-esteem. If playful engagement becomes a regular feature of the social experience, participants who previously exhibited signs of withdrawal, or physical or emotional detachment from the social environment, may start to show greater empathy in their working relationships with others in the group (Ward-Wimmer 2003). The sense of enjoyment and achievement derived from this playful engagement contributes to raised self-esteem, which is manifest in the transformation of body language, energy levels, facial expression and eye contact, and in an increased motivation to connect and communicate. Davidson et al. (2003) define a joyful life as 'an active embracing of the world' where playful engagement fosters this sense of joyfulness with corresponding benefits to physical, mental and social wellbeing (Seligman 2012).

One of the main goals in the glass studio is to use the practice of arts and crafts to expand the learning and life experience of members. Initially, there will be a period of familiarization and 'settling-in' to what is a new and potentially daunting situation. This settling-in stage is as much about the creative process and fellow artists, as the tools, machinery and studio environment. Given time, new members begin to identify with the situation and to form a growing attachment to other members of the group, to the various creative activities, and to the location. This attachment is healthy, comforting and confidence-boosting and the hope is that it will extend to the wider community through engagement and interaction with other places which then become additional sources of identification and attachment. For adults with learning disabilities, this expansion is especially important because their experience of the world can be limited to home, transportation and day-service locale (BBC 2016).

As an urban organization, Garvald Edinburgh has many social and cultural resources within easy reach, and positive learning and life-enriching attachments have been established in and around the city with, for example, the National Museum of Scotland (National Museums Scotland 2018). Museums and galleries offer a non-stigmatizing, cultural environment in which to undertake journeys of self-exploration (Colbert et al. 2013) yet, even in the enlightened art world, prejudice still exists and not all gallery spaces are welcoming to groups of adults with learning disabilities (Mordi 2015). An increase in participatory, interactive events and exhibitions may prove to be one way towards making these art spaces more accessible and user-friendly (Gross and Pitts 2016).

## Case-study: a playful odyssey

In 2018, Garvald Edinburgh chose 'Play' as the theme for an organization-wide exhibition called 'Play: Create: Relate' (Edinburgh Palette 2018). It was clear from the planning stage that, in keeping with the relational aspects of both play and social therapy, the exhibition should become a participatory endeavor. However, Bourriaud's (1998) exposition of relational art says little about the quality of the encounter or relationship that might emerge in such a participatory artistic venture (Bishop 2004). Spontaneous playfulness in a creative or learning context requires a sufficiently safe and relaxed environment in order for people to cast aside their social 'armour' or defences such that they can fully experience the freedom of creative disinhibition. Safety and social trust are prerequisites for self-expression and autonomous interaction (Maslow cited in McLeod 2018) and it was important for the experience of participation in the exhibition to be both safe and supportive, while not imposing constraints on what might happen during the artistic process. This kind of safe, open, and relaxed environment was actively fostered as a contrast to the perceived elitism typically associated with exhibition launches, which can be especially problematic for those who find new social situations difficult (McGuinness 2017).

The act of planning, creating and exhibiting a participatory art event proved to be a journey of discovery – a playful odyssey – for members of the glass studio. In order to keep the journey's route and destination as open as possible, we embarked on the process with a visual explorer exercise (Palus et al. 2014). Common themes emerging from this exercise in free association were 'feathers', 'birds' and 'flight' – with their connotations of freedom and lightness of being. These themes were developed in conversations about winged beasts, mythological creatures and Greek gods, evolving into further discussion about early humans: *Where did they come from? What were they like? Who are the gods in whose likeness we are formed?* As curiosity and interest grew, the group began designing and making glass feathers for the yet undiscovered ancestors buried in our distant past and speculation arose as to how we might imagine and give form to these 'ancient beings of light and color'. Through a process of trial-and-error, we discovered the malleable and metamorphic qualities of wax, which could be magically transformed into crystal beings of light and color. Members of the glass studio waited with great anticipation to free the first creation from its wax mould and to reveal the resulting god-like entity – but to great consternation, awe and wonder, the emergent form was a creature described by one member of the group as 'a large jelly baby'! This unexpected arrival was christened 'Baba Jello' or 'Lila', the goddess of divine play.

Who would have thought, that after millennia of speculation and curiosity about our ancient ancestry, it would transpire that our ancestors resembled a popular baby-shaped sweetie? Our Baba Jello follows in the famous footsteps of another effigy of the contemporary art world: 'Alan Measles', the teddy bear idol of Grayson Perry (2011), who appeared in his exhibition 'The Tomb of the Unknown Craftsman'.

The themes which emerged during the early stages of the creative process for the exhibition (feathers, mythology, Greek gods, early humans) contributed to an overarching motif of imagining the past and then researching ancient archaeological artefacts: clay figurines with angular, semi-abstract bodies, sometimes missing heads or feet (Sutherland 2016). These ancient treasures from around the world became our sketching source. The original intention was to create a large pair of wings constructed from glass feathers, but as members of the group made sketches from the primitive figurines they added unique characteristics derived from their own personal sketching styles, yielding an entirely new assembly of figures. During this stage of the creative process, it is important that the studio support staff do not demand realistic accuracy or perspective drawing, but encourage the unique, raw, and playful expression of the participating artists. The role of support staff is to act as facilitators: providing materials, encouragement and inspiration and enabling the flow of playful experimentation.

Self-directed expression instils the confidence to indulge in free play with material and form, with more interesting and individual results, and allows participants to act as autonomous agents in the creative process (Brookfield 2014). Autonomy in the process of creative engagement contributes to many aspects of physiological and psychological functioning typically associated with improved health status (Stuckey and Nobel 2010). When studio participants become acquainted with the idea that their unique style of expression is not only permitted but highly valued, their artistic confidence grows and is evidenced in increased autonomy and self-esteem. A positive self-image derives from this sense of achievement, pride, belonging and inclusion in a worthwhile and enriching project (Challis 2013). A robust self-image is the bedrock for the health and wellbeing not only of the individual but of the whole community.

## Sharing the creative process

At the exhibition launch of 'Play: Create: Relate', members of the glass studio had everything prepared for the visitors: a large white gallery space with works of art scattered around, on plinths, on walls, on tables and on the floor. The glass installation

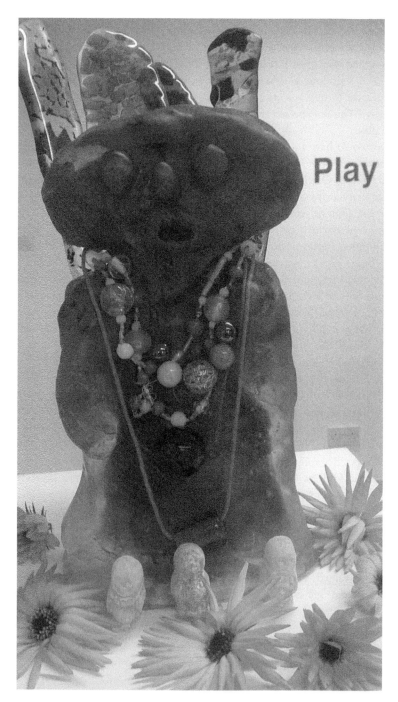

**FIGURE 4.1** *Baba Jello with Feathers* by Samantha Jones.
Source: photograph by Jane McArthur

consisted of twelve plinths, each mounted by a glass sculpture which was only partially complete. On the back of each sculpture were situated four to six holes in which were to be placed the glass feathers which would complete the figures. On another plinth, approximately 1m square, were placed a pile of 50 sand blocks/bricks, within each of which was concealed a glass feather. Tools, gloves and goggles to be used in the breaking-open of the blocks were placed close by. The plan was for visitors to the opening of the exhibition to indulge in a game of role-play, first 'playing at' archaeologist, by excavating the glass feathers and then, in the role of 'artist', choosing where to place their glass feather on the unfinished sculptures. Applying the principles of relational aesthetics, the intention was to engage with the viewing public in a different way, fostering relational qualities unobserved at more conservative exhibition openings where people typically view the artworks, meet-and-greet, and discuss in a more controlled and predictable way. It was hoped there might be an impact on how the spectators and participants would relate to the exhibition as an event, creating a different connection to the art and to each other. This reflects Gadamer's (1989) view that the act of spectatorship contributes to enhancing the being of the artwork by bringing what is at play within it to fuller realization.

The relational process can be likened to a stage-setting on which an unknown performance is about to take place. Both art and play share a 'to-and-fro' movement not tied to any specific goal other than to fulfil themselves for their own sake (ibid.).

The nature of art is essentially 'incomplete and incompletable' just as 'no one knows how the [play] will end' (Lawn 2006: 91) and this allows for a spontaneous theatricality to what unfolds, whereby the spectators respond out of their own inventiveness in an atmosphere of open play. Bakewell (cited in APPG on Arts, Health and Wellbeing 2017: 122) is quoted as saying that 'the arts need no other justification than their own intrinsic value, their capacity to lift the spirit and give us experiences of transcendental and inspirational power'. It is this power – of play, of art and of playful art – that has the potential to transform public health through the transformation of life chances.

Playful events, such as the glass studio's relational installation, allow us to explore the notions of multiple and fluid identities described by Goffman (1959). Goffman compares the self-concept to a form of role-play, purporting that 'the individual is the creative agent who decides – and who in doing so constitutes self-identity – on how to carry out such roles as well as the staging of role performances' (Elliot 2001: 32). Goffman's (1959) theory of self-concept carries important implications for those supporting adults with learning disabilities for whom the impact of social expectation may restrict the development of the self, with resultant frustration to the detriment of health and wellbeing.

## Art as installation

In their book *Installation Art in the New Millennium*, Oliveira et al. (2003) describe the art world's preoccupation with the 'theatricality' of some art projects. Installations can become 'complete immersion environments', 'theatrical spaces' in which the frame of stage and curtain is removed, and the artist and audience become as one. Those who dare to participate in 'the experience of art', experience it in a more 'open-ended manner and become authors and generators of their own meanings' (Oliveira et al. 2003). The unpredictability of the glass studio's installation for 'Play: Create: Relate' was risky in juxtaposition with the familiarity of static works of art mounted on plinths or a wall. *Would anyone want to play along? What were the barriers to the play and how would they be overcome?* It was necessary to embrace this risk and step into the realm of the unknown in order to fully inhabit the space of play.

The build-up to the exhibition, and the opening itself, proved a steep learning curve for the glass studio's group-leader. The initial intention was for a member of the glass studio (an adult with learning disabilities) to facilitate the event, but this proved to be too ambitious and those invited to assume the role of facilitator declined to do so. Working with the purpose of building self-esteem and auton-omy, and in keeping with the principles of both social therapy and relational aes-thetics, it was important to allow members to choose a level of participation with which they felt safe and comfortable (Malchiodi 2016). In the event, the active participation of those members who felt able to engage in the role-play served to motivate and encourage the participation of others.

As visitors arrived at the opening and the first person started chipping-away at a sand block, the installation developed its own momentum. Soon there was no space around the table, discarded blocks of sand piled-up on the plinth, loose sand spilled onto the floor, and some participants needed help with the excavation task; for two hours it was a non-stop frenzy of playful activity. As each glass feather was revealed then cleaned, it was added to the unfinished sculptures, thus completing the installation. The exchange of playful banter and a shared sense of fun highlighted the unifying force of play, as visitors, both adults and children, glass studio members and staff, worked towards the common goal of completing the installation. The buzz of activity, the curiosity of onlookers, the lively interaction and the positive feedback suggested that the relational aspect was successfully enacted as people set-aside day-to-day concerns and abandoned themselves to the experience of joyful, playful participation.

It was notable that the most enthusiastically spontaneous participants in the glass studio's installation were visiting children who felt no need for 'permission' to play, raising the question of how adults might be encouraged to display the same level of disinhibited playfulness.

A criticism of relational aesthetics is that its impact has been largely restricted to the contemporary art world – a unique and specific community (Bishop 2004). Broadening the appeal and accessibility of this type of experience, and learning lessons from doing so, may lead to greater insight into how to overcome social barriers to play and our own inhibitions where playfulness is concerned.

The above description and analysis of the Garvald Edinburgh exhibition, 'Play: Create: Relate', elucidates the value of participatory art, not just for the development of individual autonomy and self-esteem, but for the wider health and wellbeing of the whole community. McNiff writes that a commitment to 'expressive action that engages emotions in a direct and physical way … generate[s] creative energy as a healing force for mind, body, and spirit; and a belief that the creative imagination can find its way through out most perplexing and complex problems and conflict' (McNiff in Malchiodi 2005: ix).

## Art as meaningful experience

Artistic activity, like the pursuit of play, need not be an intellectual exercise open to only a chosen few. Participation in an interactive art installation allows for engagement on an experiential and emotional level, broadening the scope of its appeal and accessibility (Guglielmino 2007). For those with learning disabilities, the suspension of intellectual preoccupation in the practice of the arts opens-up new possibilities for creative experimentation and self-discovery and for the self-empowerment which derives from this freedom from intellectual constraints. Experiences involving creative activity generate a montage of positive feelings and associations which then transcend the moment to reach into everyday life. Gill Angell (cited in APPG on Arts, Health and Wellbeing 2017: 190), patient representative on the board at University College Hospital, is quoted as saying, 'Art allowed my soul and spirit to be nurtured and fly … [manifesting] hope, beauty and ultimately the sublime in the darkest moments'.

Cultural expression, in its many forms, has largely replaced our reliance and dependence on religious devotion (Farago 2018) and serves to elevate our lived experience to a level beyond mere physical existence, endowing it with purpose and meaning (O'Callaghan 2017). Thus, any form of self-expression which resonates with the present mood of the individual, or to which they are attuned, will have a beneficial consequence for self-esteem and for the wellbeing it generates (Gordon-Nesbitt 2015). When a creative experience represents the enactment of a personal quality in a relational connection (to other people, to the artwork, or to the gallery as a social play space), this has an impact on how the participant relates to the everyday world as a result of this unique episode in their personal narrative (Guglielmino 2007). Such an experience can provide the coordinates to help guide a person through the complex social domain which constitutes a meaningful life.

There is a deep wisdom at play in what has been described above. The concept of social capital recognizes the importance of networking for building mutually supportive relationships: 'good relationships are a major determinant of health' (White 2009). Creating opportunities for mutual support through creative self-expression and participation can bring people together in a less threatening way than everyday social encounters. This is further exemplified by the *Dragon Café* project in South London, which conceives the arts as 'nourishment' and offers a multi-dimensional menu of creative activities centered on personal narratives (APPG on Arts, Health and Wellbeing 2017: 78). The social landscape is of a challenging nature for most people, but especially so for anyone with a low sense of self-esteem (Paz et al. 2017). Play, humor and playful banter can soften the hard edges of social interaction (Palagi 2018) particularly for those who are intellectually, socially, or emotionally vulnerable. Social playfulness can be seen at work in the BBC documentary *Village of Dreams* (BBC 2018), about daily life in a Camphill community for people with learning disabilities (see www.camphill.org.uk). Playfulness imbues the relationships between the members of this community with positivity, effecting strong social bonds. Staff then pick-up on the capacity for play and channel its meandering flow into positive interactions. This use of play may be understood as an expression of emotional intelligence or 'emotional wisdom' (Chia and Saxer 2009.)

Working with adults with learning disabilities in group situations often involves personality clashes and misunderstandings; the capacity for self-reflection and emotional regulation can help to dissipate these social tensions. Emotional balance is achieved through developing an understanding of how our own attitudes and actions have an impact on those of others (Lockwood et al. 2014). Schwartz and Sharpe (2011) emphasize the role of storytelling for developing this sort of self-awareness, in that it allows for a narrative, rather than historical, understanding of our sense of self (Popova 2014). A narrative understanding arises from the play of the imagination and its significance for transformative learning. This is a common theme in the arts and underpins Steiner's integration of the creative arts in the care and education of people with additional support needs. There are also parallels with the narrative sense-making in Greek mythology (Raeburn 2004). Through the pursuit of emotional wisdom, we are helped to remain fluid in our attitudes and actions and to avoid the ossification of unhelpful approaches to life and to other people (Popova 2014). Holding on to rigid beliefs and intolerant attitudes is ultimately harmful to the self and may lead to social isolation, emotional stress and/or violence, with negative health consequences for the self and for others (Sennett 2012).

Schwartz and Sharpe (2011) describe 'practical wisdom' as the integration of emotional wisdom and the ability to cope in social situations. This 'modulated emotion' is advocated as a 'median and best course', facilitating social interactions by enabling us to do the right thing at the right time (Popova 2014) and to avoid the negative outcomes that can have an impact on our physical or mental health. Jason Bell, of the Foundation for Art and Creative Technology, confirms:

> At a time of immense emotional stress and pressure, the critical analysis skills that I had been developing making art … kept me going, giving me the weapons to fight my own demons. I have noticed a marked ability to deal with the trials and tribulations of day-to-day life, particularly, monitoring, regulating and adjusting my own behavior and my emotions.
>
> ( *APPG on Arts, Health and Wellbeing 2017: 191*)

## Conclusion

In conclusion, Steiner's advocacy for creative practices as a route to self-transformation – the discovery of the healing 'gold medicine' within (von Franz 1997: 51) – is intended to reawaken and entwine the capacities of thinking, feeling and willing which might otherwise lay dormant. Inner development through creative self-expression leads people to develop the self-confidence and associated self-esteem they need (Steiner 1997: 317). Increased autonomy and self-esteem are associated with internal motivation and self-determination and provide a tacit equilibrium central to a positive sense of self (ibid.: 314). The practice of creative arts-and-crafts has play at its core – from light-hearted playfulness to the seriousness of deep play (Ackerman 1999). From the serious play of drama, to the fun and joy of games, a readiness to embrace the playful fosters connection with place, with others, and with the 'creative, social and political' aspects of the self (Warburton 2017) – a sense of belonging to something bigger than ourselves. Steiner wrote that 'it is a sound principle to follow the path of art' (Steiner 1924), a message reinforced by contemporary research into the importance of the arts for public health: 'The arts play a vital role in creating and supporting feelings of wellbeing' and 'wellbeing is vital to our sense of who we are and to our self-worth and effectiveness' (Wiseman, cited in APPG on Arts, Health and Wellbeing 2017: 190).

## References

Ackerman, D. (1999) *Deep Play*, New York: Vintage.

APPG on Arts, Health and Wellbeing (2017) *Creative Health: The Arts for Health and Wellbeing* [The Short Report], London: All Party Parliamentary Group on Arts, Health and Wellbeing.

Bandura, A. (1978) The Self System in Reciprocal Determinism, *American Psychologist*, 33 (4): 343–358.

BBC (2016) I'm 21, Have a Learning Disability and Going Out Scares Me, retrieved from www.bbc.co.uk/newsbeat/article/35314142/im-21-have-a-learning-disability-and-going-out-scares-me (accessed 5 August 2018).

BBC (2018) *Village of Dreams* (dir. Archer J.), retrieved from www.bbc.co.uk/programmes/b0b6sthr (accessed 11 July 2018).

Bishop, C. (2004) Antagonism and Relational Aesthetics, *CUNY Academic Works*, 110: 51–79, retrieved from https://academicworks.cuny.edu/cgi/viewcontent.cgi?article=1095&context=gc_pubs (accessed 8 May 2018).

Bourriaud, N. (1998) *Relational Aesthetics*, Paris: Les Presses du reel.

Bourriaud, N. (2002) Relational Aesthetics, retrieved from www.xcult.org/medientheorie/text/Bourriaud.pdf (accessed 27 August 2018).

Brookfield, S. and James, A. (2014) *Engaging Imagination: Helping Students Become Creative and Reflective Thinkers*, San Francisco, CA: Josey-Bass.

Burt, E. and Atkinson, J. (2011) The Relationship between Quilting and Wellbeing, *Journal of Public Health*, 34(1): 54–59.

Challis, S. (2013) *How to Increase Your Self-Esteem*, London: Mind, retrieved from www.mind.org.uk/media/715750/how-to-increase-your-self-esteem-2013.pdf (accessed 4 August 2018).

Chia, M. and Saxer, D. (2009) *Emotional Wisdom: Daily Tools for Transforming Anger, Depression, and Fear*, Novato CA: New World Library.

Colbert, S., Camic, P., Cooke, A. and Springham, N. (2013) The Arts in Psychotherapy: The Art Gallery as a Resource for Recovery for People Who Have Experienced Psychosis, *The Arts in Psychotherapy*, 40: 250–256.

Cook, P. and Bellis, M. (2001) Knowing the Risk: Relationships between Risk behaviour and Health Knowledge, *Public Health*, 115(1):54–61.

Curative Education and Social Therapy Council (2018) What Is Anthroposophical Curative Education?, retrieved from www.en.khsdornach.org/What-is-anthroposophical-curat.135.0.html (accessed 5 July 2018).

Davidson, R., Kabat-Zinn, J., Schumacher, J., Rosenkranz, M., Muller, D., Santorelli, S., Urbanowski, F., Harrington, A., Bonus, K. and Sheridan, J. (2003) Alterations in Brain and Immune Function Produced by Mindfulness Meditation, *Psychosomatic Medicine*, 65: 564–570.

Deci, E. and Ryan, R. (1995) Human Autonomy: The Basis for True Self-Esteem, retrieved from www.researchgate.net/publication/232586291_Human_autonomy_The_basis_for_true_self-esteem (accessed 3 July 2018).

Dictionary.com (2018) Anthroposophy, retrieved from www.dictionary.com/browse/a nthroposophy?s=t (accessed 27 August 2018).

Doyal, L. and Gough, I. (1991) *A Theory of Human Need*, London: Macmillan.

Edinburgh Palette (2018) Play: Create: Relate, retrieved from www.edinburghpalette.co.uk/events/play-create-relate (accessed 9 July 2018).

Elliot, A. (2001) *Concepts of the Self*, Cambridge: Polity.

Farago, J. (2018) Why Museums are the New Churches, retrieved from www.bbc.com/culture/story/20150716-why-museums-are-the-new-churches (accessed 10 July 2018).

Gadamer, H.-G. (1989) *Truth and Method*, London: Sheed & Ward.

Garvald Edinburgh (2003) Principles of Social Therapy as a Basis for Our Work: A Charter for Quality, retrieved from www.garvaldedinburgh.org.uk/social-therapy-charter-3 (accessed 9 July 2018).

Goffman, E. (1959) *The Presentation of Self in Everyday Life*, New York: Doubleday.

Gordon-Nesbitt, R. (2015) *Exploring the Longitudinal Relationship Between Arts Engagement and Health*, Manchester: Arts for Health.

Gross, J. and Pitts, S. (2016) Audiences for the Contemporary Arts: Exploring Varieties of Participation across Artforms in Birmingham, UK, *Journal of Audience and Reception Studies*, 13(1): 4–23.

Guglielmino, G. (2007) *How to Look at Contemporary Art (and Like It)*, London: Umberto Allemandi and Co.

Heaney, C. (2017) What Does it Mean to Be Well?, retrieved from http://scopeblog.sta nford.edu/2017/06/19/what-does-it-mean-to-be-well (accessed 3 July 2018).

Impact Arts (2011) *Craft Café. Social Return on Investment Evaluation*, Glasgow: Social Value Lab.

Independent Living Strategy Group (2015) *Promoting People's Right to Choice and Control Under the Care Act 2014: How Are Local Authorities Performing?*, Birmingham: In Control.

James, V. (2001) *The Spirit and Art: Pictures of the Transformation of Consciousness*, Great Barrington, MA: Anthroposophic Press.

Jenson, A. (2013) Beyond the Borders: The Use of Art Participation for the Promotion of health and Well-being in Britain and Denmark, *Arts & Health*, 5(3): 204–215.

Lawn, C. (2006) *Gadamer: A Guide for the Perplexed*, London: Continuum.

Lockwood, P., Seara-Cardoso, A. and Viding, E. (2014) Emotion Regulation Moderates the Association between Empathy and Prosocial Behavior, retrieved from www.ncbi.nlm.nih.gov/pmc/articles/PMC4014517 (accessed 10 July 2018).

McGuinness, R. (2017) One in Six Britons Has Never Been to an Art Gallery, retrieved from https://uk.news.yahoo.com/one-six-britons-never-art-gallery-114847877.html?guc counter=1 (accessed 4 August 2018).

McLeod, S. A. (2018) Maslow's Hierarchy of Needs, retrieved from www.simplypsychol ogy.org/maslow.html (accessed 4 August 2018).

Malchiodi, C. (2005) *Expressive Therapies*, New York: Guilford Press.

Malchiodi, C. (2016) Expressive Arts Therapy and Windows of Tolerance, retrieved from www.psychologytoday.com/gb/blog/arts-and-health/201602/expressive-arts-therapy-a nd-windows-tolerance (accessed 24 August 2018).

Marmot, M. (2003) Autonomy, Self Esteem, and Health Are Linked Together, *British Medical Journal*, 327(7415): 574–575.

Mencap (2012) Stuck at Home: The Impact of Day Service Cuts on People with a Learning Disability, retrieved from www.bl.uk/collection-items/stuck-at-home-the-impact-of-da y-service-cuts-on-people-with-a-learning-disability# (accessed 9 July 2018).

Mordi, L. (2015) Why Museums Need to Embrace a Culture of Accessibility, retrieved from https://rereeti.wordpress.com/2015/09/09/why-museums-need-to-embrace-a-culture- of-accessibility (accessed 6 July 2018).

National Museums Scotland (2018) National Museum of Scotland, retrieved from www.nm s.ac.uk/national-museum-of-scotland (accessed 9 July 2018).

OECD (n.d.) Better Life Index, retrieved from www.oecdbetterlifeindex.org/topics/health (accessed 3 July 2018).

O'Callaghan, P. (2017) Cultural Challenges to Faith: A Reflection on the Dynamics of Modernity, *Church, Communication and Culture*, 2(1): 25–40.

Oliveira, N., Oxley, N. and Petry, M. (2003) *Installation Art in the New Millennium: The Empire of the Senses*, London: Thames & Hudson.

Palagi, E. (2018) Not Just for Fun! Social Play as a Springboard for Adult Social Competence in Human and Non-human Primates, *Behavioral Ecology and Sociobiology*, 72: 90.

Palus, C., Magellan Horth, D. and Harrison, S. (2014) About Visual Explorer, retrieved from www.ccl-explorer.org/category/visualexplorer (accessed 4 August 2018).

Paz, V., Nicolaisen-Sobesky, E., Collado, E., Horta, S., Rey, C., Rivero, M., Berriolo, P., Díaz, M., Otón, M., Pérez, A., Fernández-Theoduloz, G., Cabana, Á. and Gradin, V. B. (2017) Effect of Self-esteem on Social Interactions during the Ultimatum Game. *Psychiatry Research*, 252: 247–255.

Perry, G. (2011) *The Tomb of the Unknown Craftsman*, London: British Museum Press.

Popova, M. (2014) The Art of Practical Wisdom, retrieved from www.brainpickings.org/ 2014/04/14/practical-wisdom-barry-schwartz (accessed 10 June 2018).

Public Broadcasting Service (2018) In the Mix: Self-Expression, Self-Esteem … Around the World, retrieved from www.pbs.org/inthemix/shows/show_selfexpression.html (accessed 3 July 2018).

Public Health England (2018) Learning Disabilities: Applying All Our Health, retrieved from www.gov.uk/government/publications/learning-disability-applying-all-our-health/lea rning-disabilities-applying-all-our-health (accessed 4 July 2018).

Raeburn, D. (2004), *Metamorphoses: A New Verse Translation*, London: Penguin.

Schwartz, B. and Sharpe, K. (2011) *Practical Wisdom: Doing the Right Thing at the Right Time*, New York: Penguin Group.

Seligman, M. (2012) *Authentic Happiness: Using the New Positive Psychology to Realize Your Potential for Lasting Fulfilment*, New York: Free Press.

Sennett, R. (2003) *Respect in a World of Inequality*, New York: Norton.

Sennett, R. (2008) Labours of Love, *The Guardian*, 2 February, retrieved from www.theguardia n.com/books/2008/feb/02/featuresreviews.guardianreview14 (accessed 21 August 2018).

Sennett, R. (2012) *Together: The Rituals, Pleasures and Politics of Cooperation*, London: Penguin.

Sigman, A. (2015) Practically Minded. The Benefits and Mechanisms Associated with a Practical Skills-Based Curriculum, retrieved from http://thefieldcentre.org.uk/wp-con tent/uploads/2015/11/Practically-Minded-2015.pdf (accessed 14 August 2018).

Steiner, R. (1997) *An Outline of Esoteric Science*, New York: Anthroposophic Press.

Steiner, R. (1924) Lecture Nine. Abnormal Paths into the Spiritual World and Their Transformation, retrieved from https://wn.rsarchive.org/Lectures/GA243/English/ RSP1969/19240820p01.html (accessed 13 August 2018).

Stuckey, H. and Nobel, J. (2010) The Connection Between Art, Healing, and Public Health: A Review of Current Literature, *American Journal of Public Health*, 100(2): 254–263.

Sutherland, A. (2016) Mysterious Figurine of Mythical Individual Dates Back to Egypt's Naqada Culture 4400–3000 BC, retrieved from www.ancientpages.com/2016/09/25/figurine-m ythical-individual-dates-back-egypts-naqada-culture-4400-3000-bc (accessed 10 August 2018).

Tate (2018) Relational Aesthetics, retrieved from www.tate.org.uk/art/art-terms/r/relationa l-aesthetics (accessed 5 July 2018).

Tite, R., Kavanagh, S. and Novais, C. (2016) *Everyone's An Artist (or At Least They Should Be): How Creativity Gives You the Edge in Everything You Do*, New York: Collins.

Von Franz, M. (1997) *Alchemical Active Imagination*, Boston, MA: Shambhala.

Warburton, A. (2017) Playmakers, retrieved from www.craftscouncil.org.uk/articles/playma kers (accessed 15 May 2018).

Ward-Wimmer, D. (2003) The Healing Potential of Adults at Play, in C. E. Schaefer (ed.), *Play Therapy with Adults*, 1–11, New York: Wiley.

White, M. (2009) *Arts Development in Community Health: A Social Tonic*, Florida: CRC Press.

Wigham, S. and Emerson, E. (2015) Trauma and Life Events in Adults with Intellectual Disability, *Current Developmental Disorders Reports*, 2(2): 93–99.

Wilson, N., Jaques, H., Johnson, A. and Brotherton, M. (2017) From Social Exclusion to Supported Inclusion: Adults with Intellectual Disability Discuss Their Lived Experiences of a Structured Social Group, *Journal of Applied Research in Intellectual Disabilities*, 30: 847–858.

Womack, S. (2005) Backlash Growing against Healthy Eating Campaigns of 'Do-Gooders', *The Telegraph*, 27 April, retrieved from www.telegraph.co.uk/news/uknews/1488753/Backla sh-growing-against-healthy-eating-campaigns-of-do-gooders.html (accessed 8 July 2018).

# 5

## PLAYING TOGETHER

### The art and the science of relationships

*Julia Whitaker and Alison Tonkin*

## Introduction

The need to form enduring social relationships lies at the heart of what it means to be human (Hawkley and Cacioppo 2010). Research professor Brene Brown is quoted as saying: 'A deep sense of love and belonging is an irresistible need of all people. We are biologically, cognitively, physically, and spiritually wired to love, to be loved, and to belong' (Brown cited in Seppala 2012). The drive to form relationships is universal: evident in all cultures and across social groups (Deci and Ryan 2000) and theorists from Freud (1930), Maslow (1968) and Bowlby (1969) to Bowen (1985) and Baumeister (1995) have recognized the human need for relatedness as a primary motivator for social behavior.

Research now shows that relationship quality is directly linked to specific areas of public health concern such as child poverty, infant attachment, mental health, obesity, alcohol/substance misuse, cardiovascular disease and dementia (Meier 2013). Furthermore, the quality of social relationships has also been directly linked to mortality in a manner 'comparable with well-established risk factors for mortality such as smoking and alcohol consumption and [exceeding] the influence of other risk factors such as physical inactivity and obesity' (ibid.: 2).

The impact of our relationships reaches beyond the quality of interpersonal connections and personal health profiles; it applies equally to the individual's connections with the wider social systems in which they operate and the connections between these systems themselves. The application of systems theory to the study of public health acknowledges the contextual nature of relationships – their 'social ecology' (Marjoribanks 2016) – and recognizes that interpersonal relationships exist in symbiosis with wider relationships – with school, work, community and public services. This relational approach demands a conceptual shift from 'atomism to holism', from an individualistic model in which the individual is the sole agent of their destiny, to one in which 'the socially embodied individual – located in the context of their inter-relationships and social practices – is placed centre-stage' (ibid.: 10).

In this chapter, an adapted interpretation of Bronfenbrenner's (2009) ecological model has been used to differentiate the impact of relationship quality on health and wellbeing at different stages in the life-course and how a relational approach broadens the scope for playful intervention.

## Contextualizing ecological approaches

The use of ecological approaches to explore the multiple contexts that influence and connect the behavioral mechanisms underlying health-related behaviors is becoming more common (Moran et al. 2016). The traditional focus of scholarly activity on individualistic mechanisms, such as beliefs and attitudes, is changing and 'researchers are expanding their scope of inquiry to include more macro-level contexts such as family, peers, neighborhood, as well as the broader culture or society' (ibid.: 135).

Bronfenbrenner (1977) proposed that the progression of human development throughout life is, in part, a consequence of the interaction between the developing human and the dynamic environment in which the individual lives. This includes the immediate setting, which has a direct impact on the individual, but also the wider formal and informal social contexts that surround the setting, which have an indirect influence on human development (Bronfenbrenner 1977). A pictorial representation of the individual within the wider social context (shown in Figure 5.1) can be useful as a means of exploring social networks and the

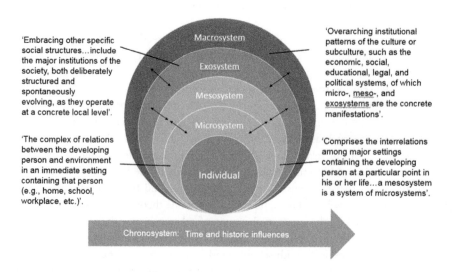

**FIGURE 5.1** Pictorial representation of Bronfenbrenner's ecological environment. Source: adapted from Bronfenbrenner (1977: 514)

level of 'connectedness within an individual's environment' (Fenge 2017: 56). Bronfenbrenner (1977: 514) conceptualized the environment 'topologically as a nested arrangement of structures, each contained within the next', which Nelson and Lund (2017) have similarly described as the individual 'nestled in concentric circles of influential systems'.

One important feature of an ecological systems approach is the assumption that all factors within and across the systems are 'interrelated and mutually influential', from the level of the individual through to the macro-level (Moran et al. 2016: 135). This enables a more holistic scoping of the potential for positive health change, incorporating the 'interpersonal, community and societal contexts in which individuals live' (ibid.: 136).

## The individual

With the individual as the traditional focus of policy and strategic planning, factors such as biological and physical attributes, personality traits, attitudes, beliefs and self-efficacy have dominated interventions and academic research in the public health arena (Blue et al. 2014). Over 40 years ago, Bronfenbrenner (1977: 525) observed that placing emphasis on individual traits, with limited reference to context, 'has generated a curiously broken trajectory of knowledge that has a brave beginning [childhood], a sad ending [decline in older age], and an empty middle', due to the paucity of research undertaken in the intervening years. Today, public health interventions still focus on the individual but there is parallel acknowledgement of the context in which the individual lives, and a broader scope in terms of age is now factored into interventions. For example, Public Health England (2016) has launched One You, which identifies that 'living healthily in midlife can double your chances of being healthy at 70 and beyond'. In the news story linked to the release of One You in 2016, Professor Sir Muir Gray, clinical advisor for the campaign, stated, 'Although it has been customary to blame people for their "lifestyle" we now appreciate that we need to take into account the environmental pressures that make it difficult to make healthy choices, having to sit 8 hours a day at work for example, and then drive an hour home' (ibid.). Emphasis has also been placed on society's involvement in the campaign, the object being to make One You visible 'in every community, on every high street, in local health services, on websites and on social media. We want everyone across the country to know that it is never too late to get your health back on track' (ibid.). Perhaps one of the most noticeable differences within the One You campaign, is the emphasis on health and fitness as a means of maintaining relationships with loved ones, with the implication that living longer and in better health will generate more quality time with family and friends. 'Staying happy' is also highlighted, supporting the view that good health incorporates the emotional wellbeing which allows people 'to do the things [they] love and make [them] happy, like seeing friends or taking part in activities or hobbies' (Public Health England 2018).

## The microsystem

The microsystem includes direct influencers on the individual's development, encompassing the individual's relationships and interactions with his or her immediate surroundings such as family, school, neighborhood, or care environment (Lohrmann 2008).

Research evidence from the ACE Study (Centers for Disease Control and Prevention 2014) identifies stable family relationships as one of the key protective factors against adversity in childhood. Chapter 6 discusses the importance of early attachment for the development of positive relationships throughout life, and advocates for play as crucial to the development of this attachment relationship. In Chapter 7 play and playfulness are endorsed as a counterbalance to the everyday demands and stresses of modern family life. The concept of play as a key contributor to psycho-social resilience acknowledges that the capacity to adapt to change, and to thrive in the face of difficulty and challenge, derives not solely from individual qualities but also from the individual's experience of family, social networks and neighborhood.

A study by Brinker and Cheruvu (2017) found that social and emotional support can mitigate against the psychological distress associated with the experience of adverse childhood experiences and recommends interventions designed to promote social and emotional support in order to alleviate the mental health burden. Folostina et al. (2015) have demonstrated how play and drama sessions can positively influence the level of resilience in children at risk of poverty and social exclusion: 'Through art and play, a child in a special needs situation can explore the physical and social environment, address past and current emotional issues, can create a role and reach a state of satisfaction from imaginary events.' (ibid.: 2362). However, the capabilities that foster resilience can be strengthened at any age: opportunities for regular physical exercise, stress-relieving activities such as music and art, innovative use of children's toys (Figure 5.2), and games that actively promote cognitive function and emotional regulation can improve the ability of adults to adapt to, cope with, and even avoid adversity throughout life.

## The mesosystem

Mesosystems connect two or more of the systems in which the child, parent and family live. It is important that mesosystems represent consistent and complementary approaches to lifestyle values and priorities in order for the fulfilment of the potential of optimal health (Australian Research Alliance for Children and Youth and the Australian Institute of Health and Welfare 2010). The role of *culture* is 'indispensable and important for addressing inequalities and inequities in health as well as for facilitating culture-sensitive health communication strategies that will ultimately close the gap on the social determinants of health and risk' (Iwelunmor and Airhihenbuwa 2017).

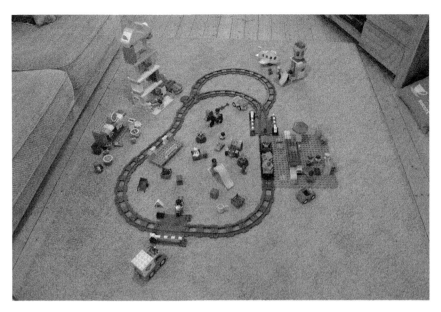

**FIGURE 5.2** Rigby Town – Duplo date night.
Source: James Rigby (Rigby Town made by Megan and James Rigby)

Every place and every community has its own culture, a common narrative about how and where its people live, work and play. There exist within and between these *cultures of place* 'shared and sometimes contested values, local traditions, behaviors and drivers for change' (Reeves 2017), and the challenge for public health is to match its efforts to these cultural variables. The British Academy's 'Where We Live Now' project found that, 'At a time when, it is clear, many people feel increasingly disconnected from those who make decisions', the culture of place 'offers a means of reconnection, more sensitive and appropriate policy-making, and better outcomes in terms of our individual and societal wellbeing' (British Academy 2017: 2) Public health improvement is about exploiting every possibility of change through innovation, action, adaptation and experiment (Reeves 2017).

Until their demolition in 2015, the infamous Red Road Flats in the northeast of Glasgow, Scotland, were an icon of the social and economic deprivation associated with failed housing schemes of the 1960s. The flats were a structural reflection of the neglect, damage and hopelessness which had come to characterize the social decline of a whole community. Yet, at the heart of this same broken community, the Red Road Women's Center represented a haven where local women could find relief from the social isolation associated with living in high-rise housing in an area of deprivation. It was from the Women's Center that the Women@Play group hatched in 2004, as part of an art project undertaken in partnership with Glasgow's Gallery of Modern Art (Hollows 2007). Women@Play drew on the parallels between the broken environment and the women's experiences of violence, and their decision to share their ideas about this connection through 'the simple act of play' (Bruce et al. 2007: 50). Each week, the Red Road women chose an activity which they played in the space in front of the flats, inviting others 'out to play' in a collective act of strength and unity. The zenith of the project was a self-organized, community-wide event which involved over 100 women wearing red scarves and coming together below the flats to form the shape of 'The Labyrinth of Life', an apt metaphor for their own journeys through a complex social landscape (Bruce et al. 2007). The women decorated the scarves with messages and images related to their own personal life maps, which had acquired new meanings as they were re-visited in the company of others.

Research confirms that people's perceptions of the physical quality of their social environment correlate with their experience of loneliness: people who have a negative perception of their neighborhood, use fewer local amenities, and know fewer people in the community, are also more likely to be lonely (Kearns et al. 2015). The Localism Act (Communities and Local Government Committee 2011) advocated 'the devolution of powers to citizens and grass roots organisations', essentially opening 'the way to a bigger role for the participatory arts, which are delivered locally and often regarded as a means of individual and community empowerment' (APPG on Arts, Health and Wellbeing 2017). The Red Road women's project reinforces the principle that place-based approaches to public health, which align with the local culture, are the most likely to meet the unique needs of the communities they serve (Ham and Alderwick 2015). Relationships built on common ground are relationships built on trust and mutual under-standing, and arts engagement – which often involves casual social contact at a local level – is regularly cited as a forum for building trust (APPG on Arts, Health and Wellbeing 2017: 79).

## The exosystem

The exosystem includes peers and family social networks, neighborhood and community services such as school and the workplace. Generally influenced by local politics, the exosystem defines the larger social system which indirectly impacts individual development, health and wellbeing – and access to play. The exosystem is particularly important when considering the lived experience of loneliness (Fenge 2017).

Loneliness, or perceived social isolation, can affect anyone and the nature of loneliness differs according to the life stage when it occurs (Griffin 2010). Humans are social creatures and they rely 'on a safe, secure social surround to survive and thrive' (Hawkley and Cacioppo 2010: 218). However, Monbiot (2014) bleakly states that 'for the most social of creatures, the mammalian bee, there's no such thing now as society. This will be our downfall.' Perhaps the economic burden of loneliness on 'individual, collective and societal health … is a prompt to revitalize our communities, and better integrate their members' (Griffin 2010: 33). The exosystem has the potential to promote collective efficacy, identify community norms and develop community health capacity, all of which are being used to combat loneliness at a local level (Moran et al. 2016).

Loneliness is essentially a natural emotional state which is embedded in human evolution (Griffin 2010). Cacioppo (cited Klinenberg 2018) suggests that 'an occasional and transitory feeling of loneliness can be healthy and productive. It's a biological signal to ourselves that we need to build stronger social bonds'. In this context, Monbiot (2014) suggests 'there are palliatives, clever and delightful schemes like Men in Sheds and Walking Football developed by charities' that provide opportunities for social engagement on a regular basis and which are fun and enjoyable for those who are able to take part.

Griffin (2010) identifies chronic loneliness as a much more difficult problem to solve, suggesting that a two-pronged attack is necessary, namely providing interventions that make people feel less isolated as well as promoting the importance of links with other people. Play and playful endeavors provide genuine opportunities for social engagement at both individual and societal levels. Simple activities such as talking to neighbors and colleagues can make a difference to an individual's perceived social isolation. Modest, relatively inexpensive acts of societal engagement are performed daily by volunteers in the community. For example, in Yorkshire, England, once a month on a Sunday (known to be the loneliest day of the week), people who live alone are being invited to afternoon tea parties hosted in a family home, enabling them to enjoy the social comradery of being part of a family (Rutter 2017).

The arts also have a role to play in supporting social engagement. Cutler states:

> [A] broad range of community activities [can] help stave off loneliness – from faith groups to leisure, from the arts to fitness and outdoor pursuits, to education and learning, to hobbies and clubs … There can be enormous social benefits – creating a 'look forward to' moment in the week, bringing people together and fostering new friendships.
>
> *(Cutler 2012)*

New technologies have changed the way people work, play and interact and they now offer a range of new ways to bring people together, bridging cultural, generational and geographic divides (Griffin 2010). Social media platforms, such as Facebook and Twitter, and interactive gaming, such as Pokémon Go (discussed in more detail in Chapter 11), are the millennial generation's equivalents of gossiping over the garden fence or the parish dance.

## The macrosystem

The macrosystem represents our relationship to the cultural values, traditions and policies which impact on lifestyle choices and opportunities, and consequently on health. These systems include social groupings, religious affiliations and ethnic identity. Ongoing sociocultural change has an inevitable impact on our attitudes and behaviors with corresponding implications for our understanding of public health and wellbeing.

Play lies at the heart of all our relationships, from the mutual mirroring of mother and infant and the real and imaginary friendships of childhood, to the romantic dalliances of youth and our life-long enthusiasms. The place of play in the macrosystem is ever-changing, reflecting the evolution of societal values, attitudes and priorities and the policy responses to the pattern of this evolution. The meaning of 'play' as a construct in contemporary society is widely debated (e.g. Elkind 2001) and the status of play in the 21st century goes beyond individual connectedness to reflect four key variables: 'changing generational traits and preferences, educational reform, the growing social dimension of play and the rise of game mechanics to drive wide-spread behavior change in society' (Gauntlett et al. 2010: 5).

In 2002, the LEGO Learning Institute initiated an empirical study of parental values, beliefs, and attitudes towards their children's use of time and the balance between scheduled activities and opportunities for free play (LEGO Learning Institute 2002). The study found that parents think they should try to create a balance in their children's lives between free play and scheduled activities. Parents know that time for free play is crucial to children and acknowledge that when children are engaged in play they also learn and grow. However, they also feel a duty to prepare their children for adult working life and believe that the best way to do this is to enrol their children in organized activities with an educational element. The study concluded that 'free play is squeezed in favour of "goal oriented" and "real world conforming" activities' (LEGO Learning Institute 2002: 4). It also identified significant cross-cultural differences in the value ascribed to free play: 32 per cent of UK parents felt that children's free time is often 'wasted' compared with just 5 per cent of Japanese parents. 52 per cent of the parent sample regarded time spent doing 'nothing in particular' was wasted time, while this 'free time' was relatively more appreciated by parents over 35 years of age with a high level of educational attainment and a higher income level. Furthermore, the definitions of what constitutes play seem to have expanded to include interaction with electronic media (television, video games, internet) and even shopping – 38 per cent of the parent sample regarded shopping as a form of play. Attitudes to play and how we engage in play behavior clearly cannot be understood in isolation from the constantly changing sociocultural environment, including rapid technological developments and an increasing focus on consumption as a leisure activity.

Marjoribanks (2016) argues that central government has a responsibility to take a proactive approach to drive local action to respond positively to societal change, and to foster the conditions necessary for people to adapt and thrive. He cites the Australian government's 1999 National Families Strategy as an example of a successful national approach to supporting family relationships. The strategy's aim of preventing family breakdown by developing effective early intervention, focused specifically on 'provision of marriage and relationship support services such as relationship education, parenting education, relationship counselling, and mediation' (Marjoribanks 2016: 23). This collaborative response to public priorities was based on common values ('family' and 'relationships') and a stated commitment to change. If we are to realize the vision of a strong and healthy society, based on positive relationships between individuals and between systems, we need to identify and acknowledge the challenges we face and to accept our collective responsibility to openly explore developmental opportunities, including a renewed recognition of play as a force for good.

When Bronfenbrenner (1977) conceptualized the original ecological model, environmental influencers referred to 'concrete manifestations' which were tangible and 'real'. In the early 1980s, when the modern internet was invented, a virtual world of intangible influential systems was created which has radically changed the ways in which we interact with our sociocultural environment. The Internet Revolution is perhaps the most far-reaching historical revolution of modern times, responsible for re-shaping communications, business, and politics, and changing the way in which people conduct their everyday lives (see Chapter 11). While the internet offers huge benefits in terms of information exchange and social connectivity, there has emerged a growing awareness of its negative consequences in terms of the invasion of personal privacy and the risk of human exploitation – particularly in relation to children and young people (Vittana.org n.d.).

The problem of cyber bullying – which takes place through chat rooms, instant messaging, social media, and other forms of digital electronic communication – is now recognized as a major area of public health concern (National Academies of Sciences, Engineering, and Medicine 2016) because of its association with a wide range of physical and mental health issues, as well as with alcohol and substance abuse and increased violence in adolescence and adulthood (Dhar 2013).

There are numerous innovative attempts to tackle the problem of cyber bullying (Foley 2016) – many themselves online initiatives. In the UK, the charity *ChildLine* exploits the possibilities offered by the internet to connect with its target group, alongside its core business providing free, confidential services for anyone under 19 years of age. ChildLine offers help and advice on 'anything – from abuse and bullying to exam stress and relationships' through phone, e-mail and one-to-one chats with a counsellor (ChildLine 2018a). The charity has a strong digital platform, including a virtual Toolbox which includes games, creative activities, mood-boosting suggestions and advice videos. It states: 'However you're feeling, it can be great to express yourself and do things you enjoy' (ChildLine 2018b). The Creative Corner of the website invites browsers to 'write down [their] stories, poems and thoughts' using message boards with different themes, while the Art Box encourages users to express their feelings in words or drawings (ChildLine 2018c).

The Fabulous Four Activity Diary (BBC Headroom, cited in ChildLine 2018d) promotes the scheduling of activities that are known to enhance wellbeing, but which are often suspended when problems arise. These include:

- pleasurable activities;
- activities which give you a sense of achievement;
- activities which make you physically active; and
- social activities.

The activity diary encourages users to practice a balance of activities from each group, varying them from day to day, to find a pattern that suits their own needs and lifestyle (BBC Headroom, cited in ChildLine 2018d). The remedial benefits of playful pursuits derive from the fact that they are freely chosen, reinforcing a sense of agency when life feels out of control (Sutton-Smith 2003).

One example of a more dynamically playful approach is that on offer by the Take Away Theatre Company in the UK (see www.takeawaytheatre.co.uk). This touring theater group specializes in anti-bullying performances for schools, and their highly acclaimed interactive production, *Hope*, combines music, drama and humor to deliver a serious message – much in the same way that children have always used play to enact matters of serious personal concern. 'Play-acting' reflects the pretend play of early childhood in that it allows for the safe expression of both positive and negative feelings, the modulation of affect, and the ability to integrate emotion with cognition (Kaufman 2012). The concept of 'theory of mind' (Jenkins and Astington 2000) – the awareness that one's thoughts may differ from those of another and that one is capable of adopting a variety of perspectives – is closely related to imaginative play and is utilized by the Take Away Theatre Company to challenge perceptions of a bullying scenario. Research demonstrates that a school environment in which pretend games are a feature of the curriculum or play-time (recess) nurtures the development of independent thinking, problem-solving, decision-making and creative and imaginative skills (Ashiabi 2007) – the very life skills which build the social and emotional resilience necessary to thrive in an internet-dominated world.

## The chronosystem

The chronosystem sits outside the nested structure of influential systems and represents a 'time-based dimension that influences the operation of all levels of the ecological systems' (Johnson 2008). It refers to the time dimensions of the individual over the course of the lifespan, as well as to the socio-historical framing of the macrosystem which also changes over time (ibid.).

The world population is aging – with significant implications for public health (Lancet Public Health 2017). In 2015, it was calculated that seven per cent of the global population were aged over 65 and it is estimated that this proportion will increase to 17 per cent by the year 2050 (He et al. 2016). In the UK, the number of over 65s has already reached 18 per cent of the total population (Office for National Statistics 2017) while 15 per cent of US citizens are over 65 (US Census Bureau 2017). In 2011, more than a quarter of a million (291,000) of the over-65s in England and Wales were living in care homes, representing 3.2 per cent of the total population within this age-group (Office for National Statistics 2014). As people live longer, it is important that they have access to appropriate health and care services and a recognition of the importance of play and playfulness in older age can ensure that these services enable older people to live a life of quality for all their days, regardless of physical, cognitive or social impairment (Dunn et al. 2013).

Increased social interaction is key to improved physical and mental health in old age, as highlighted in the Channel 4 documentary *Old People's Home for 4 Year Olds* (Channel 4 Television Corporation 2018) which found that a group of care home residents experienced measurable improvements in mood, mobility and memory after spending just six weeks with a group of visiting pre-schoolers. The growing interest in the concept of intergenerational care as a way of purposefully bringing together different generations to share experiences of mutual benefit, locates play and playfulness center stage (e.g. The Intergenerational Care Project, Australia; The Intergenerational Learning Center, Seattle, USA). Generations United's 'Tried and True' guide to successful intergenerational activities (Jarrott 2007) emphasize the play concept of 'process over performance' and the need to remove any expectation of pre-determined outcomes. Durand (2007) explains: 'being flexible about where activities may lead gives children and adults a chance to build relationships of discovery'.

In the UK, Eden Project Communities (see www.edenprojectcommunities.com) has recognized that 63 per cent of grandparents now look after grandchildren on a regular basis with the introduction of their 'Deep Roots, New Shoots' programme (Tolley 2017) which aims to provide shared playful experiences across the generational divide. Intergenerational play offers older people an investment in the future through engagement with the young, and encourages both children and adults to explore new challenges with mutual benefits for physical and cognitive health and a consequently enhanced quality of life.

## Conclusion

Life starts and ends with a relationship: from the infant's first gaze into the mother's eyes to the final hand-hold at life's end, who we are and how we live are determined by our connections to the people and places around us. There is now a wealth of evidence to show that these social connections – our relationships – are crucial not only to our physical and mental health but to the health of the societies in which we live. Positive social connections form the underlay for the prosocial behaviors – trust, empathy and cooperation – on which healthy communities are built. A relational approach to public health opens the door to an appreciation of the potential of play as a mediator in this process. Whether as a means of learning, healing, helping or just being neighborly, play nurtures and sustains our connections with each other and with the world around us. Csikszentmihalyi (1992) writes, 'A community should be judged good … if it offers people a chance to enjoy as many aspects of their lives as possible, while allowing them to develop their potential in the pursuit of ever greater challenges' (Csikszentmihalyi 1992: 191).

## References

APPG on Arts, Health and Wellbeing (2017) *Creative Health: The Arts for Health and Wellbeing* [The Short Report], London: All Party Parliamentary Group on Arts, Health and Wellbeing.

Ashiabi, G. (2007) Play in the Preschool Classroom: Its Socioemotional Significance and the Teacher's Role in Play, *Early Childhood Education Journal*, 35(2): 199–207.

Australian Research Alliance for Children and Youth and the Australian Institute of Health and Welfare (2010) *Conceptualisation of Social and Emotional Wellbeing for Children and Young People, and Policy Implications*, Sydney: Australian Research Alliance for Children and Youth.

Baumeister, R. (1995) The Need to Belong: Desire for Interpersonal Attachments as a Fundamental Human Motivation, *Psychological Bulletin*, 117(3): 497–529.

Blue, S., Shove, E., Carmona, C. and Kelly, M. (2014) Theories of Practice and Public Health: Understanding (Un)healthy Practices, *Critical Public Health*, 26(1): 36–50.

Bowen, M. (1985) *Family Therapy in Clinical Practice*, New York: Jason Aronson.

Bowlby, J. (1969) *Attachment and Loss: Vol. 1. Attachment*, New York: Basic Books.

Brinker, J. and Cheruvu, V. (2017) Social and Emotional Support as a Protective Factor against Current Depression among Individuals with Adverse Childhood Experiences, *Preventative Medicine Reports*, 5: 127–133.

British Academy (2017) *The Way We Live Now: Making the Case for Place-Based Policy*, London: British Academy.

Bronfenbrenner, U. (1977) Toward an Experimental Ecology of Human Development, *American Psychologist*, 32(7): 513–531.

Bronfenbrenner, U. (2009) *The Ecology of Human Development: Experiments by Nature and Design*, Cambridge, MA: Harvard University Press.

Bruce, K., Harman, B., Hollows, V. and Watson, A. (2007) *Towards an Engaged Gallery*, Glasgow: Culture and Sport Glasgow (Galleries).

Centers for Disease Control and Prevention (2014) ACE Study, retrieved from https://web. archive.org/web/20151227092712/www.cdc.gov/violenceprevention/acestudy/index. html (accessed 19 March 2018).

Channel 4 Television Corporation (2014) Old People's Home for Four Year Olds, retrieved from www.channel4.com/programmes/old-peoples-home-for-4-year-olds (accessed 27 March 2018).

ChildLine (2018a) About ChildLine, retrieved from www.childline.org.uk/about/about-ch ildline (accessed 3 April 2018).

ChildLine (2018b) Toolbox: Games, retrieved from www.childline.org.uk/toolbox/gam es/#filter (accessed 3 April 2018).

ChildLine (2018c) Creative Corner, retrieved from www.childline.org.uk/get-support/m essage-boards/boards/?boardid=81&roomid=-1 (accessed 3 April 2018).

ChildLine (2018d) Activity Scheduling: The Fabulous Four, retrieved from www.childline. org.uk/globalassets/info-and-advice/your-feelings/feelings-and-emotions/depression-a nd-feeling-sad/activity-plan-the-fabulous-four.pdf (accessed 4 April 2018).

Communities and Local Government Committee (2011) *Third Report: Localism*, London: Communities and Local Government Committee.

Csikszentmihalyi, M. (1992) *Flow: The Psychology of Happiness*, London: Random House.

Cutler, D. (2012) *Tackling Loneliness in Older Age – The Role of the Arts*, London: Baring Foundation and Campaign for Loneliness.

Dhar, M. (2013) Bullying Increasingly Seen as a Public Health Issue, retrieved from www. huffingtonpost.com/2013/11/08/bullying-public-healthissue_n_4241468.html (accessed 26 March 2018).

Deci, E. and Ryan, R. (2000) The What and Why of Goal Pursuits: Human Needs and the Self-Determination of Behavior, *Psychological Inquiry*, 11: 227–268.

Dunn, J., Balfour, M., Moyle, W., Cooke, M., Martin, K., Crystal, C. and Yen, A. (2013) Playfully Engaging People Living with Dementia: Searching for Yum Cha Moments, *International Journal of Play*, 2(3): 174–186.

Durand, S. (2007) You're Never Too Old To Play: Intergenerational Learning Programs, retrieved from www.geteduca.com/blog/intergenerational-learning (accessed 27 March 2018).

Elkind, D. (2001) *The Hurried Child. Growing Up Too Fast Too Soon*, New York: Perseus Publishing.

Fenge, L. (2017) Loneliness, Well-being and Scam Involvement, in L. Fenge, S. Lee and K. Brown (eds), *Safeguarding Adults: Scamming and Mental Capacity*, 53–64, London: Sage.

Foley, M. (2016) Cyberbullying Is A Serious Public Health Problem, Says Report, But These 5 Organizations Hope To Stop Online Harassment In Its Tracks, retrieved from www.bustle.com/articles/161064-cyberbullying-is-a-serious-public-health-problem-sa ys-report-but-these-5-organizations-hope-to-stop (accessed 26 March 2018).

Folostina, R., Tudorache, L., Michel, T., Erzsebet, B., Agheana, V. and Hocaoglu, H. (2015) Using Play and Drama in Developing Resilience in Children at Risk, *Procedia – Social and Behavioral Sciences*, 197: 2362–2368.

Freud, S. (1930) *Civilization and its Discontents* (trans. J. Riviere). London: Hogarth Press.

Gauntlett, D., Ackermann, A., Whitebread, D., Wolbers, T. and Weckstro, C. (2010) *The Future of Play. Defining the Role and Value of Play in the 21st Century*. Billund: The Institute.

Griffin, J. (2010) *The Lonely Society?* London: Mental Health Foundation.

Ham, C. and Alderwick, H. (2015) *Place-Based Systems of Care: A Way Forward for the NHS in England*, London: The King's Fund.

Hawkley, L. and Cacioppo, J. (2010) Loneliness Matters: A Theoretical and Empirical Review of Consequences and Mechanisms, *Annals of Behavioral Medicine*, 40(2): 218–227.

He, W., Goodkind, D. and Kowal, P. (2016) *An Aging World 2015*, Washington, DC: US Census Bureau.

Hollows, V. (2007) Giving Elbow Room: Contemporary Art and Human Rights, in K. Bruce, B. Harman, V. Hollows and A. Watson (eds), *Towards an Engaged Gallery*, 7–22. Glasgow: Culture and Sport Glasgow (Galleries).

Iwelunmor, J. and Airhihenbuwa, C. (2017) Culture, a Social Determinant of Health and Risk: Considerations for Health and Risk Messaging, retrieved from http://communica tion.oxfordre.com/view/10.1093/acrefore/9780190228613.001.0001/acre fore-9780190228613-e-221 (accessed 3 April 2018).

Jarrott, S. (2007) *Tried and True: A Guide to Successful Intergenerational Activities at Shared Site Programs*, Washington, DC: Generations United.

Jenkins, J. and Astington, J. (2000) Theory of Mind and Social Behavior: Casual Models Tested in a Longitudinal Study, *Merrill-Palmer Quarterly*, 46: 203–220.

Johnson, E. (2008) Ecological Systems and Complexity Theory: Toward an Alternative Model of Accountability in Education, *Complicity: An International Journal of Complexity and Education*, 5(1): 1–10.

Kaufman, S. B. (2012) The Need for Pretend Play in Child Development: Imaginative Play is a Vital Component to Normal Child Development, retrieved from www.psychology today.com/us/blog/beautiful-minds/201203/the-need-pretend-play-in-child-developm ent(accessed 26 March 2018).

Kearns, A., Whitley, E., Tannahill, C. and Ellaway, A. (2015) 'Lonesome Town'? Is Lone-liness Association with the Residential Environment, Including Housing and Neigh-bourhood Factors? *Journal of Community Psychology*, 43(7): 849–867.

Klinenberg, E. (2018) Is Loneliness a Health Epidemic?, *The New York Times*, 9 February, retrieved from www.nytimes.com/2018/02/09/opinion/sunday/loneliness-health.html (accessed 4 April 2018).

Lancet Public Health (2017) Ageing: a 21st Century Public Health Challenge?, *The Lancet Public Health*, 2(7).

LEGO Learning Institute (2002) *Time for Playful Learning? A Cross-Cultural Study of Parental Values and Attitudes toward Children's Time for Play*, Billund, Denmark: LEGO Learning Institute.

Lohrmann, D. (2008) A Complementary Ecological Model of the Coordinated School Health Program, *Public Health Reports*, 123(6): 695–703.

Marjoribanks, D. (2016) *All Together Now*, London: Relate.

Maslow, A. (1968) *Toward a Psychology of Being*, New York: Van Nostrand.

Meier, R. (2013) *Relationships: The Missing Link in Public Health*, London: The Relationships Alliance.

Monbiot, G. (2014) The Age of Loneliness Is Killing Us, *The Guardian*, 14 October, retrieved from www.theguardian.com/commentisfree/2014/oct/14/age-of-loneliness-killing-us (accessed 4 April 2018).

Moran, B., Frank, L., Zhao, N., Gonzalez, C., Thainiyom, P., Murphy, S. and Ball-Rokeach, S. (2016) An Argument for Ecological Research and Intervention in Health Communication, *Journal of Health Communication*, 21(2): 135–138.

National Academies of Sciences, Engineering, and Medicine(2016) *Preventing Bullying Through Science, Policy, and Practice*, Washington, DC: The National Academies Press.

Nelson, J. and Lund, E. (2017) Bronfenbrenner's Theoretical Framework Adapted to Women with Disabilities Experiencing Intimate Partner Violence, in A. J. Johnson, J. Nelson and E. Lund (eds), *Religion, Disability, and Interpersonal Violence*, 11–23. Berlin: Springer International Publishing.

Office for National Statistics (2014) Changes in the Older Resident Care Home Population between 2001 and 2011, retrieved from www.ons.gov.uk/peoplepopulationandcomm unity/birthsdeathsandmarriages/ageing/articles/changesintheolderresidentcarehomepopula tionbetween2001and2011/2014-08-01 (accessed 26 March 2018).

Office for National Statistics (2017) Overview of the UK Population: July 2017, retrieved from www.ons.gov.uk/peoplepopulationandcommunity/populationandmigration/popula tionestimates/articles/overviewoftheukpopulation/july2017 (accessed 27 March 2018).

Public Health England (2016) PHE Launches One You, retrieved from www.gov.uk/gov ernment/news/phe-launches-one-you (accessed 4 April 2018).

Public Health England (2018) One You: Checking, retrieved from www.nhs.uk/oneyou/ checking#0RDEAQ4yVsYohjuW.97 (accessed 4 April 2018).

Reeves, D. (2017) *Under the Skin: Stories that Explore the Culture of Place*, Edinburgh: Grant Thornton.

Rutter, T. (2017) 'There's a Taboo around Loneliness': Meet the People Tackling the Epidemic, *The Guardian*, 26 January, retrieved from www.theguardian.com/careers/ 2017/jan/26/theres-a-taboo-around-loneliness-meet-the-people-tackling-the-epidemic (accessed 4 April 2018).

Tolley, E. (2017) Intergenerational Play, retrieved from www.edenprojectcommunities. com/blog/intergenerational-play (accessed 26 March 2018).

Seppala, E. (2012) Social Connection Improves Health, Well-Being & Longevity, retrieved from www.psychologytoday.com/blog/feeling-it/201208/connect-thrive (accessed 19 March 2018).

Sutton-Smith, B. (2003) Play as a Parody of Emotional Vulnerability, in J. L. Roopnarine (ed.), *Play and Educational Theory and Practice. Play and Culture Studies, Vol. 5*, 3–17, Westport, CT: Praeger.

US Census Bureau (2017) Facts for Features: Older Americans Month: May 2017, retrieved from www.census.gov/newsroom/facts-for-features/2017/cb17-ff08.html (accessed 27 March 2018).

Vittana.org (n.d.) The Pros and Cons of the Internet, retrieved from https://vittana.org/ 12-pros-and-cons-of-internet (accessed 26 March 2018).

# 6

# PLAY, ATTACHMENT AND THE EMPATHY–EQUITY CONNECTION

*Julia Whitaker*

## Introduction

This chapter explores the connection between the human instinct to play (Bekoff 2017) and the development of the social empathy necessary for the creation of a healthy society (Bazalgette 2017). Empathy – 'the ability to stand in somebody else's shoes and see the world through their eyes' (President Barack Obama, cited in New York Times 2007) – is a prerequisite for the mutual respect, understanding and compassionate action necessary for the creation of a universal 'culture of health' (Lavizzo-Mourey 2018). The concept of *social* empathy (Segal 2011) extends this definition to include 'the ability to more deeply understand people by perceiving or experiencing their life situations and as a result gain insight into structural inequalities and disparities'. The development of social empathy is of relevance to public health because it advocates policies 'that address disparities and support social and economic justice for all people' (ibid.).

The health of any society is affected by a wide range of influences, and the collaborative approach espoused in the UK government's Five Year Forward View (NHS England et al. 2014) calls for action and alignment across a number of different levels, from public institutions to local communities and individuals (Alderwick et al. 2015). A revisiting of the concept of attachment, in the light of what is now known about the importance of relationships for lifelong health and wellbeing, raises the profile of play as a catalyst in the development of empathy and how this impinges on health and happiness in the social context.

## Health equity as a human right

A public health approach to health equity reflects government aspirations to eliminate social and health differences that are 'unnecessary, avoidable, and unfair' (Whitehead 1991). This bold ambition is underpinned by the Universal Declaration of Human

Rights (1948) and its stated recognition 'of the inherent dignity and of the equal and inalienable rights of all members of the human family [as] the foundation of freedom, justice and peace in the world' (United Nations n.d.). Health equity is a fundamental public health concern, not only because it is essential to an individual's wellbeing and to their ability to be fully engaged in society, but because a healthy society is necessary for social, economic and political stability (Braveman et al. 2011). However, seventy years after the publication of the UN Declaration of Human Rights, it remains the case that a worldview based on 'freedom, justice and peace' is stubbornly undermined by inequities in the health and wellbeing of the global family (Goh 2017). There exists almost a ten-year differential in life expectancy between children born in the wealthiest and the poorest regions of the United Kingdom (Office for National Statistics n.d.), while a child born in Africa is six times more likely to die in the first year of life than a child born in Europe (World Health Organization 2018a). In the US, there is little evidence of any progress towards eliminating health disparities by race or socio-economic status (Voelker 2008).

Public health efforts to address such inequalities require a smorgasbord approach which acknowledges the interrelated influences on the health and wellbeing of the whole population, and which incorporates contributions from 'science, knowledge and intelligence, advocacy, partnerships, and the delivery of specialist public health services' (Public Health England 2016). Raising the status of empathy on the public health agenda is key to making the shift from a 'self-interest frame' of mind to a 'common-interest frame', wherein health priorities are decided by a concern for both ourselves *and* for others (Crompton 2010). Public health interventions which address the social concomitants of health pay heed to the psycho-social nature of health differentials (Friedl 2009) while acknowledging the life-long significance of early experience and the role of playful interaction in establishing the *empathy instinct* (Bazalgette 2017).

Empathy has been variously conceptualized, with definitions including: 'to know another person's inner experience' (Buie 1981: 282) and 'to accurately perceive, interpret and respond to the emotional signals of others' (Preston and de Waal 2002). It is an important aspect of human development because it has been associated with emotional wellbeing, positive interpersonal relationships, and overall 'life success' (Mehrabian 2000). Research in the field of cognitive neuroscience has identified the neurobiology of empathy (e.g. Iacoboni 2008), while attachment theory advocates the critical role of nurture, or lived experience, for its development (e.g. Masur 2009). The association between play and attachment is well-established (e.g. Ginsberg 2007) and complementary research into the neurological and psycho-social impact of early experience recognizes a role for play in the development of social empathy and its significance for health equity and consequently for public health.

## From attachment to empathy

Human survival, like that of all mammals, depends on our ability to connect with others of our species. This connectivity determines not only our physical survival but also the nature of our relationships with each other and with the social context of our lives. de Waal (2001: 21) writes that reliance on others is essential to our survival: 'Every human life cycle includes stages at which we either depend on others (when we are young, old or sick) or others depend on us (when we care for the young, old or sick).' This notion of mutual dependency is mirrored in the public health concept of the *healthy setting* (World Health Organization 2018b), which advocates the co-creation of physical and social environments and community resources which enable people to mutually support each other in the fulfilment of their lived potential. Commitment to others, emotional sensitivity to their situation, and an understanding of what kind of help they might need, define the very essence of humanity (de Waal 2001) and these are traits which emerge from that first point of connection: the bond between parent and child.

Few models of human development have attained greater universal acceptance than *attachment theory* which expounds the cruciality of early infant bonding to psycho-social wellbeing in adult life. The pioneering work of John Bowlby (1969) explained variations in adult behavior and mental health in terms of early childhood experiences and, most specifically, the relationship between mother and child – a relationship regarded as the prototype for all future social relationships. The enduring influence of attachment theory is now reinforced by neurological research into the way the brain processes emotion (Schore 2000).

Trevarthen and Aitken's (2001) exploration of the links between brain development, infant communication and emotional health suggests that very young infants rapidly develop proto-cultural intelligence through interacting with other people, including in teasing fun play. Trevarthen (2014) maintains that babies are motivated by a desire for connection and companionship (including playfulness and fun) and that the development of *intersubjectivity* (shared understanding or mutual empathy) is supported by the adult caregiver's responsiveness to the baby's initiative. He identifies 'playful human respect' as the key to this emotional synchrony. Feldman (2007) showed that the degree of synchrony between mothers and babies during the first year, was directly associated with measures of empathy in childhood and adolescence. The more that mothers and babies matched and influenced each other's behaviors during face-to-face play during infancy, the greater the expressed empathy in mother-child interactions during middle childhood and adolescence. The child who is engaged in a respectful, playful interaction recognizes that their own feelings are shared by another and comes to realize that their own emotionally motivated actions can have an influence on the other person. McDonald and Messinger (2011) suggest that it is this realization which promotes the sense of potency necessary for acting on a desire to help others. Longitudinal studies have shown that young children whose parents demonstrate warmth towards them also tend to show greater empathy towards others (e.g. Zhou et al. 2002). In summary:

it seems that parents who provide a warm, positive environment for their children, and who provide a model for being sensitive to others' needs and emotions through synchronous interactions with their child and talking about emotions with their child are most likely to have more empathic children.

*(McDonald and Messinger 2011)*

An array of creative initiatives illustrates the role of play and playfulness in supporting the evolution from early attachment to this capacity for empathy or 'fellow feeling'. The positive power of engagement with the creative arts resides in their capacity to offer an insight into the human condition – to understand and to feel understood. Booth (1988: 1) quotes the artist Andrew Harrison: 'A work of art … is a bridge between one mind and another … it's a primary way in which people create and exchange meaning.'

The Creative Families project (South London Gallery 2015) is one which demonstrates the positive association between creative play and attachment. Participation in artist-led projects which explored parenting, motherhood, collaborative art-making, skill-sharing and typography resulted in increased parental confidence and self-determination, with positive repercussions for mother-child attachment and the emotional and social development of the child. The Music and Motherhood project (Royal College of Music 2018) is another example of a playful initiative which fosters the synchronous interactions found to underlie the development of empathy through shared experience. During a ten-week period, groups of mothers attended weekly music workshops in which they listened to, learnt, wrote and sang songs with their babies and initial findings suggest that singing stimulates a positive emotional response in mothers, promoting mother-child bonding with lifelong consequences for future relationships.

Attachment theory offers a valuable framework for understanding how we connect with each other and how we develop close, mutually supportive, relationships as resources for coping with life's challenges (Lopez and Brennan 2000; Mallinckrodt 2000). Neff and McGehee (2010) make a parallel link between self-compassion and the development of empathy. Self-compassion is defined as an adaptive way of relating to the self in the face of personal inadequacies or difficult life circumstances (ibid.) and is learned through parental modeling. When family experiences are consistently caring and supportive, the child develops a compassionate perception of themselves, with implications for both their personal wellbeing and for the development of social empathy (Stevens and Woodruff 2018).

The development of self-compassion may also be nurtured through engagement in the creative arts and creative play projects, as demonstrated by the many initiatives designed to improve the social and emotional wellbeing of children in hospital. The illness of a child challenges family relationships and functioning on many levels, and playful interaction through engagement with the arts can preserve and promote the parent–child bond which underlies the development of personal wellbeing and empathic attitudes and behaviors. One representative example is the *Magical Journeys* collaboration (Adam 2016) between the National Portrait Gallery and five Central London hospitals, which offered creative arts opportunities to the families of children with long-term health conditions. Active participation in the appreciation and practice of the visual arts has a positive impact on health and wellbeing in that it has been shown to positively affect mood, feelings of self-worth and a general sense of wellbeing (Royal Society for Public Health 2013) and the evaluation of the Magical Journeys initiative reinforces the impact and value of projects of this kind. Patients and their families were given the opportunity to share stress-free and pleasurable times, co-creating positive and creative experiences and memories of their time in hospital. The project evaluation showed that the children experienced physical, cognitive, social and emotional benefits including improved coping with their hospital treatments, indicative of the development of self-compassion.

Opportunities for creative play, and for active engagement with the arts, support the attachment relationship because they involve an active, sensory-based dynamic between parent and child which includes matching, mirroring, role-play, witness, demonstration and sharing – the building blocks of empathy (Malchiodi 2013). Creative, play-based interventions may, therefore, also be helpful in repairing and reshaping negative attachment patterns. Repetitive, experiential, and self-rewarding experiences which are shared with a benevolent other, are crucial for overcoming disrupted attachment through the development of a positive sense of self in relation to the other and of the trust which is crucial for the formation of meaningful relationships (Perry 2009). A study by Cobbett (2016) has established the potential benefits of creative art therapies for children and young people with a history of insecure attachments. Over the course of a year, a group of children who took part in a combination of music, drama and arts programmes showed significant improvement in social, emotional and behavioral development, in comparison with a control group.

The observed benefits of creative activities for the attachment process, for self-compassion and for the development of empathy are now being understood in terms of their effects on the brain. Baron-Cohen (2011) has identified key regions of the brain involved in understanding both the self and others, reinforcing the widely held view that we need to have the experience of being understood and cared about ourselves, before we can empathize with others (Nierenberg 2017). In the words of Gottschall (2013: 67), referring to the power of the imagination, 'The constant firing of our neurons in response to fictional stimuli strengthens and redefines neural pathways that lead to skilful navigation of life's problems.'

Parents with a negative attachment history, or who face specific parental challenges, have been shown to benefit from help to bond with their own children across three pivotal domains: knowledge and understanding of child development; sensitive and responsive interactional skills; and time and opportunity for mutually satisfying play with their child (Grossman and Grossman 2018). Five to Thrive is an example of a flexible learning programme for parents and early years practitioners which is designed to enhance awareness of five key activities for healthy brain development in babies – respond, cuddle, relax, play, talk. Described as the 'building blocks for a healthy brain', these are also key components of the processes of attachment and attunement (Pettitt, 2015). Five to Thrive has been shown to nurture attachment through increasing parents' knowledge and understanding of how they can best support their child's emotional development, while boosting parental confidence in their own ability to meet their child's nurture needs.

Positive attachment is a vital, but not sufficient, prerequisite for the development of empathy and the positive relationships which are necessary for personal happiness and optimal engagement with the social group. Grossman et al. (2008) stress that 'secure exploration must complement secure attachments so that children can successfully meet the many challenges posed by their social relationships'. Play offers the perfect conduit both for attachment and for exploration: play, particularly free exploratory play, promotes the flexibility of thought and behavior required for self-regulation and the ability to cope with challenge and change. The sense of mastery derived from imaginative, creative play develops resilience and adaptability and contributes to confidence and self-esteem. The balance between attachment and exploration, first demonstrated in the laboratory setting by Ainsworth and Bell (1970), has been much debated, and it is now accepted (e.g. Grossman et al. 2008) that the nature and extent of the child's exploratory play is a good indicator not only of the security of the attachment bond but of a child's social and emotional development.

The child who forms strong attachments at the start of life develops a robust sense of themselves as a unique person, worthy of care and attention and capable of managing their own emotions. Positive parental engagement and modeling through playful interaction generates the trust which underlies the capacity for forming and maintaining positive relationships based on empathy and cooperation. 'Playful activities can reduce stress, strengthen attachment, and solve behavior problems while bringing laughter and joy to [the parents] and the children' (Solter, 2013: 3).

## Play, happiness and health

The synchronous interactions observed between well-attached babies and their mothers are reflected in the courtship behavior of young lovers (Maister and Tsakiris 2016) and in the mutual understanding characteristic of long-married couples (Guerrero and Floyd 2006). De Waal (2001) writes, 'When I see synchrony and mimicry – whether it concerns yawning, laughing, dancing or aping – I see social connection and bonding.'

It seems likely that the quality of attachments in adulthood may account in part for individual differences in wellbeing (McDonald and Messinger 2011). Diener and Seligman (2002) found that having close inter-personal relationships contributes significantly to happiness, suggesting a link between the ability to build and maintain relationships and subjective wellbeing. There is now sound evidence that happiness also has a beneficial impact on physiological health; on the cardiovascular and immune systems, on hormone and inflammation levels, and on the rate of wound-healing (Diener et al. 2017). Epel and Blackburn (2017) have exposed the link between subjective wellbeing and the length of our telomeres – the chromosome caps which determine how fast cells age and die – and neuroscientific research now suggests 'a direct tie from psychological well-being to aging and health at the cellular level' (Diener et al. 2017). Ongoing research into so-called *superagers* – those aged 80 and over whose sharp mental faculties defy their advanced years – highlights the contribution made by having satisfying, high-quality relationships. The superagers are notable 'for their optimism, resilience, and perseverance – as well as active and engaged lifestyles, marked by pursuits like travel, reading, and positive social relationships' (Dockrill 2018). It seems that a 'habit of play' (Fahey 2015), supported by close personal relationships, affects more than just quality of life, but also the way in which our brains age.

Robinson (2017) has written of the 'play = happiness' equation:

> When it comes to beefing up your happiness, it's hard to do better than engaged play. Not only does it align you with your deepest needs and deliver fun in the moment, but the social component of play is a huge predictor of increased daily well-being.

Studies show that play is the closest reflection of the 'true self' (Waterman 2015). Activities which are self-chosen and intrinsically motivated, and which include elements of 'personal expressiveness' (*play*), satisfy core self-determination needs such as autonomy and competence and contribute to the integration of the different parts of the self and thus to optimal psychological functioning. Csikszentmihalyi's (2008) concept of 'flow' echoes Maslow's (1943) view that it is full involvement in the moment which produces optimal experiences and Neulinger (1981:17) describes the passionate pursuit of play as 'a quality of action or even a dimension of life … fundamental to our species' nature'.

Graham (2008) asserts that it is inequality, rather than economic poverty, which has a negative effect on human development and on our personal experience of happiness and consequently on our health and wellbeing. Studies have shown that both physical and mental health are better in societies where income is more equally distributed and suggest that this relationship is most likely mediated by the impact of inequality on social relationships and by the level of status differentiation in different societies (Pickett and Wilkinson 2010). A public health approach based around social empathy is one which acknowledges the attachment relationship as one of the psycho-social determinants of health and which recognizes playful interaction as an instrument of connectivity.

## Attachment and empathy at the root of resilience

Human development is a lifelong sequence of interrelated experiences which connect brain, body and environment in a constant, reciprocal process of adaptation and change (Edelman 2007). Attachment at the start of life represents the bedrock of this developmental journey, since it is in the context of the attachment relationship that the neurological and psycho-social potential for trust, confidence and empathy are established.

Mounting research evidence of the life-long effects of adverse childhood experiences (ACE's) has reinforced awareness of the impact of psycho-social stress at the start of life on health and wellbeing throughout the lifespan (e.g. Mersky et al. 2013; Hughes et al. 2017). A report by Public Health England (2017) quotes Friedl (2009: iii) as saying, 'whilst psychosocial stress is not the only route through which disadvantage affects outcomes, it does appear to be pivotal'. Secure attachment experiences are positively associated with self-compassion, personal wellbeing and empathy for others (Wei et al. 2011) and positive attachments which provide the experience of feeling cared for, connected, and emotionally contained (Neff and McGehee 2010) contribute not only to individual resilience and wellbeing but to an empathic connection with the wider social group.

Play has been described as 'childhood's inborn tool to build resilience' (Ginsburg and Jablow 2014). Through their play, children learn to adapt to and shape their physical and psycho-social environments, and play is recognized as a protective shield against the potentially damaging effects of early social and emotional disadvantage. Research into the benefits of spending time in the natural environment has raised awareness of the importance of outdoor play for all children – and adults – with projects such as Nature Nurture (see https://naturenurture.org.uk) in Scotland promoting resilience 'by combining free-play and nurturing interactions in natural environments'. The MOVE project in Eastern Europe (Terre des Hommes 2012) promoted the playing of traditional games as a means of building the life-skills necessary for self-protection, resilience and greater self-esteem. In Nigeria, UNESCO (2018) are engaged in a collaborative play initiative designed to promote young children's resilience and their potential to foster a peaceful and sustainable future through play.

A resilience model emphasizes protective factors in the face of risk and adversity and focuses on strengths in the child, family and community which can be nurtured and supported by public policy (Evans and Pinnock, 2007). The United Nations Children's Fund report titled *The State of the World's Children 2012: Children in an Urban World* (UNICEF 2012) highlights the Dutch concept of *Woonerf* ('living street' or 'home zone') as an example of a public health practice with the potential to enhance the holistic health and resilience of children and their families through the creation of public play spaces, inviting further discussion on 'the balance ... between public and private space and between individual and collective well-being' (Gill 2006). This is addressed more fully in Chapter 12.

Killian (2015) makes the case that resilience derives more from the contexts, systems and relationships with which a person identifies than from individual attributes. Public health policies which focus on early intervention for identified target, or 'at risk', groups have been criticized for their emphasis on the individual as a 'social investment' rather than concern for universal wellbeing in the present, and for overlooking the importance of children's social and cultural relationships (Evans and Pinnock, 2007). Lester and Russell (2008) purport that children's development and wellbeing cannot be understood in isolation from their social context. This chapter represents an attempt to examine how the nature and extent of our connectivity within our social group, and with society generally, are determined by the development of the social empathy which finds its origins in early attachment experiences.

## Conclusion

The human capacity for empathy is an important public health consideration because it fosters positive attitudes and behavior towards others and facilitates the social interactions crucial for the formation of positive relationships. McDonald and Messinger (2011) propose that empathy also motivates the desire to help others, upon which rests the public health concept of the compassionate community. Almost everyone has the capacity for empathy, but how that capacity evolves depends on our earliest experiences of attachment, which are both formed and reformed through playful interaction. If we are to ensure that the art and science of empathy are reflected in public health policy, we need also to build on the evidence for play as a crucial mediator in this relationship.

## References

Adam, S. (2016) *The National Portrait Gallery Hospital Arts Programme Evaluation Report*, London: National Portrait Gallery.

Ainsworth, M. and Bell, S. (1970) Attachment, Exploration, and Separation: Illustrated by the Behavior of One-Year-Olds in a Strange Situation, *Child Development*, 41(1): 49–67.

Alderwick, H., Ham, C. and Buck, D. (2015) *Population Health Systems: Going Beyond Integrated Care*, London: The Kings Fund.

Baron-Cohen, S. (2011) *Zero Degrees of Empathy: A New Theory of Human Cruelty*, London: Allen Lane.

Bazalgette, P. (2017) *The Empathy Instinct*, London: John Murray.

Bekoff, M. (2017) Wild Justice, Cooperation and Fair Play, in R. Sussman, (ed.), *The Origins and Nature of Sociality*, 53–80, London: Routledge.

Booth, W. (1988) *The Company We Keep: An Ethics of Fiction*, Berkeley, CA: University of California Press.

Bowlby, J. (1969) *Attachment and Loss, Vol. 1: Loss*, New York: Basic Books.

Braveman, P., Kumanyika, S., Fielding, J., LaVeist, T., Borrell, L., Manderscheid, R. and Troutman, A. (2011) Health Disparities and Health Equity: The Issue Is Justice, *Journal of the American Psychoanalytic Association*, 101(Suppl 1): 149–155.

Buie, D. (1981) Empathy: Its Nature and Limitations, *Journal of the American Psychoanalytic Association*, 29(2): 281–307.

Cobbett, S. (2016) Reaching the Hard to Reach: Quantitative and Qualitative Evaluation of School-Based Arts Therapies with Young People with Social, Emotional and behavioural Difficulties, *Emotional and behavioural Difficulties*, 21(4): 403–415.

Crompton, T. (2010) *Common Cause: The Case for Working with Our Cultural Values*, Godalming: World Wildlife Fund UK.

Csikszentmihalyi, M. (2008) *Flow: The Psychology of Optimal Experience*, New York: Harper Perennial.

De Waal, F. (2001) *The Age of Empathy: Nature's Lessons for a Kinder Society*, London: Souvenir Press.

Diener, E. and Seligman, M. (2002) Very Happy People, *Psychological Science*, 13(1): 81–84.

Diener, E., Pressman, S., Hunter, J. and Delgadillo-Chase, D. (2017) If, Why, and When Subjective Well-Being Influences Health, and Future Needed Research, *Applied Psychology Health and Well-Being*, 9: 133–167.

Dockrill, P. (2018) *Scientists Are Revealing The Brain Difference That Turns Some People Into 'Superagers'*, retrieved from www.sciencealert.com/less-than-5-superagers-what-they-have-in-common-elderly-sharp-cognitive (accessed 21 February 2018).

Edelman, G. (2007) *Second Nature: Brain Science and Human Knowledge*, New Haven, CT: Yale University Press.

Epel, E. and Blackburn, E. (2017) *The Telomere Effect: A Revolutionary Approach to Living Younger, Healthier, Longer*, London: Orion.

Evans, R. and Pinnock, K. (2007) Promoting Resilience and Protective Factors in the Children's Fund: Supporting Children and Young People's Pathways towards Social Inclusion?, *Journal of Children and Poverty*, 13(1): 21–36.

Fahey, R., 2015, The Habit of Play, retrieved from https://usplaycoalition.org/the-habit-of-play (accessed 21 February 2018).

Feldman, R. (2007) Mother–Infant Synchrony and the Development of Moral Orientation in Childhood and Adolescence: Direct and Indirect Mechanisms of Developmental Continuity, *American Journal of Orthopsychiatry*, 77: 582–597.

Friedl, L. (2009) *Mental Health, Resilience and Inequalities*, Geneva: World Health Organization.

GillT. (2006) Home zones in the UK: History, Policy and Impact on Children and Youth, *Children, Youth and Environments*, 16: 90–103.

Ginsberg, A. (2007) The Importance of Play in Promoting Healthy Child Development and Maintaining Strong Parent-Child Bonds, *Pediatrics*, 119(1): 182–191.

Ginsburg, K. and Jablow, M. (2014) *Building Resilience in Children and Teens. Giving Kids Roots and Wings*, Itasca, IL: American Academy of Pediatrics.

Goh, S. (2017) Immorality of Inaction on Inequality, retrieved from www.bmj.com/content/356/bmj.j556/rr-8 (accessed 25 January 2018).

Gottschall, J. (2013) *The Storytelling Animal: How Stories Make Us Human*, Boston, MA: Houghton Mifflin Harcourt.

Graham, C. (2008) Happiness and Health: Lessons and Questions for Public Policy. Health Affairs, retrieved from www.researchgate.net/profile/Carol_Graham/publication/5670831_Happiness_And_Health_Lessons_And_Questions_For_Public_Policy/links/0c960530b6a9dbdcb8000000.pdf (accessed 7 February 2018).

Grossmann, K., Grossmann, K., Kindler, H. and Zimmermann, P. (2008) A Wider View of Attachment and Exploration: The Influence of Mothers and Fathers on the Development of Psychological Security from Infancy to Young Adulthood, in J. Cassidy and P. Shaver (eds), *Handbook of Attachment: Theory, Research, and Clinical Applications*, 2nd edition, 348–365, New York: Guilford.

GrossmannK. and GrossmannK. (2018) The Impact of Attachment to Mother and Father and Sensitive Support of Exploration at an Early Age on Children's Psychosocial Development through Young Adulthood, retrieved from www.child-encyclopedia.com/sites/default/files/textes-experts/en/567/the-impact-of-attachment-to-mother-and-father-and-sensitive-support-of-exploration-at-an-early-ageon-childrens-psychosocial-development-through-young-adulthood.pdf (accessed 8 February 2018).

Guerrero, L. and Floyd, K. (2006) *Nonverbal Communication in Close Relationships*, London: Routledge.

Hughes, K., Bellis, M., Hardcastle, K., Sethi, D., Butchart, A., Mikton, C., Jones, L. and Dunne, M. (2017) The Effect of Multiple Adverse Childhood Experiences on Health: A Systematic Review and Meta-analysis, *Lancet Public Health*, 2: e356–366.

Iacoboni, M. (2008) *Mirroring People: The New Science of How We Connect with Others*, New York: Farrar, Straus and Giroux.

Killian, K. (2015) What is Resilience? Placing a Buzz Word in Social Context, retrieved from www.psychologytoday.com/blog/intersections/201509/what-is-resilience-placing-buzz-word-in-social-context (accessed 27 February 2018).

Lavizzo-Mourey, L. (2018) Building a Culture of Health in America, retrieved from www.youtube.com/watch?v=h6N8D70yOqk (accessed 1 February 2018).

Lester, S. and Russell, W. (2008) *Play for a Change: Play, Policy and Practice: A Review of Contemporary Perspectives: Summary Report*, London: National Children's Bureau.

Lopez, F. and Brennan, K. (2000) Dynamic Processes Underlying Adult Attachment Organization: Toward an Attachment Theoretical Perspective on the Healthy and Effective Self, *Journal of Counseling Psychology*, 47: 283–301.

McDonald, N. and Messinger, D. (2011) The Development of Empathy: How, When, and Why, in A. Acerbi, J. Lombo and L. Sanguineti (eds), *Free Will, Emotions and Moral Actions: Philosophy and Neuroscience in Dialogue*, IF Press, retrieved from https://pdfs.semanticscholar.org/fdd6/748d36caed021a7698f6c40d4f0a0e728d4e.pdf (accessed 1 February 2018).

Maister, L. and Tsakiris, M. (2016) Intimate Imitation: Automatic Motor Imitation in Romantic Relationships, *Cognition*, 152: 108–113.

Malchiodi, C. (2013) Creative Art Therapy and Attachment Work: Part Two, retrieved from www.psychologytoday.com/blog/arts-and-health/201309/creative-art-therapy-and-atta chment-work-part-two (accessed 22 February 2018).

Mallinckrodt, B. (2000) Attachment, Social Competencies, Social Support and Interpersonal Process in Psychotherapy, *Psychotherapy Research*, 10: 239–266.

Maslow, A. (1943) A Theory of Human Motivation, *Psychological Review*, 50: 370–396.

Masur, C. (2009) Parent–Infant Psychotherapy, *Journal of the American Psychoanalytic Association*, 57(2): 467–473.

Mehrabian, A. (2000) Beyond IQ: Broad-Based Measurement of Individual Success Potential or 'Emotional Intelligence', *Genetic, Social, and General Psychology Monographs*, 126: 133–239.

Mersky, J., TopitzesJ., and ReynoldsA. (2013) Impacts of Adverse Childhood Experiences on Health, Mental Health, and Substance Use in Early Adulthood: a Cohort Study of an Urban, Minority Sample in the US, *Child Abuse and Neglect*, 37(11):917–925.

Neff, K. and McGehee, P. (2010) Self-compassion and Psychological Resilience among Adolescents and Young Adults, *Self and Identity*, 9(3): 225–240.

Neulinger, J. (1981) *The Psychology of Leisure*, Minneapolis, MN: C. C. Thomas.

New York Times (2007) The Democratic Presidential Debate on MSNBC, *The New York Times*, 26 September, retrieved from www.nytimes.com/2007/09/26/us/politics/26DEBATE-TRANSCRIPT.html (accessed 28 February 2018).

NHS England, Care Quality Commission, Health Education England, Monitor, Public Health England and NHS Trust Development Authority (2014) *NHS Five Year Forward View*, London: NHS England, retrieved from www.england.nhs.uk/ourwork/futurenhs (accessed 28 February 2018).

Nierenberg, C. (2017) Knowing Yourself: How to Improve Your Understanding of Others, retrieved from www.livescience.com/59349-knowing-yourself-helps-your-understand-others.html (accessed 26 February 2017).

Office for National Statistics (n.d.) Life Expectancies, retrieved from www.ons.gov.uk/peop lepopulationandcommunity/birthsdeathsandmarriages/lifeexpectancies (accessed 25 January 2018).

Perry, B. (2009) Examining Child Maltreatment through a Neurodevelopmental Lens, *Journal of Trauma and Loss*, 14, 240–255.

Pettitt, B., 2015, *Bringing Five to Thrive Alive*, Ilford: Barnardos.

Pickett, K. and Wilkinson, R. (2010) Inequality: An Underacknowledged Source of Mental Illness and Distress, *British Journal of Psychiatry*, 197: 426–428.

PrestonS. and de WaalF. (2002) Empathy: Its Ultimate and Proximate Bases, *behavioural and Brain Sciences*, 25: 1–71.

Public Health England (2016) *Local Health and Care Planning: Menu of Preventative Interventions*, London: Public Health England.

Public Health England (2017) *Psychosocial Pathways and Health Outcomes: Informing Action on Health Inequalities*, London: Public Health England.

Robinson, J. (2017) The Key to Happiness: A Taboo for Adults?, retrieved from www.huffingtonpost.com/joe-robinson/why-is-the-key-source-of-_b_809719.html (accessed 7 February 2018).

Royal College of Music (2018) Music and Motherhood, retrieved from www.rcm.ac.uk/research/projects/musicandmotherhood (accessed 20 February 2018).

Royal Society for Public Health (2013) Arts, Health and Wellbeing Beyond the Millennium: How Far Have We Come and Where Do We Want to Go?, retrieved from www.rsph.org.uk/about-us/news/arts–health-and-wellbeing-beyond-the-millennium–how-far-have-we-come-in-15-years-.html (accessed 20 February 2018).

Schore, A. (2000) Attachment and the Regulation of the Right Brain, *Attachment and Human Development*, 2(1): 23–47.

SegalE. (2011) Social Empathy: A Model Built on Empathy, Contextual Understanding, and Social Responsibility That Promotes Social Justice, *Journal of Social Service Research*, 37(3): 266–277.

Solter, A. (2013) *Attachment Play: How to Solve Children's Behavior Problems with Play, Laughter, and Connection*, Goleta, CA: Shining Star Press.

South London Gallery (2015) *Making it Together: An Evaluative Study of Creative Families, an Arts and Mental Health Partnership between the South London Gallery and Parental Mental Health Team*, London: South London Gallery.

Stevens, L. and Woodruff, C. (eds) (2018) *The Neuroscience of Empathy, Compassion, and Self-Compassion*, Cambridge, MA: Academic Press.

Terre des Hommes (2012) Traditional Games for Child Protection, retrieved from https://childhub.org/sites/default/files/2012_Traditional%20Games_EN.pdf (accessed 5 March 2018).

Trevarthen, C. (2014) Pride and Shame in Adventures of Companionship: Primary Aesthetic and Moral Values for Human Meaning and Their Importance in Early Development, retrieved from www.psychevisual.com/Video_by_Colwyn_Trevarthen_on_Pride_and_shame_in_adventures_of_companionship_Primary_aesthetic_and_moral_values_for_human_meaning_and_their_importance_in_early_development.html (accessed 23 January 2018).

Trevarthen, C. and Aitken, K. (2001) Infant Intersubjectivity: Research, Theory, and Clinical Applications, *Journal of Child Psychology and Psychiatry*, 42(1): 3–48.

UNESCO (2018) China and Africa Share Experiences on Play and Resilience Project, retrieved from www.unesco.org/new/en/harare/about-this-office/single-view/news/china_and_africa_share_experiences_on_play_and_resilience_pr (accessed 26 February 2018).

UNICEF (2012) *The State of the World's Children 2012: Children in an Urban World*, New York: UNICEF.

United Nations (n.d.) Universal Declaration of Human Rights, retrieved from www.un.org/en/universal-declaration-human-rights (accessed 25 January 2018).

VoelkerR. (2008) Decades of Work to Reduce Disparities in Health Care Produce Limited Success, *Journal of the American Medical Association*, 299(12): 1411–1413.

Waterman, A. (2015) What Does It Mean to Engage in Identity Exploration and to Hold Identity Commitments? A Methodological Critique of Multidimensional Measures for the Study of Identity Processes, *Identity*, 15(4): 309–349.

Wei, M., Liao, K. Y.-H., Ku, T.-Y. and Shaffe, P. (2011) Attachment, Self-Compassion, Empathy, and Subjective Well-Being Among College Students and Community Adults, *Journal of Personality*, 79: 1.

World Health Organization (2018a) Infant Mortality, retrieved from www.who.int/gho/child_health/mortality/neonatal_infant_text/en (accessed 25 January 2018).

World Health Organization (2018b) Healthy Settings, retrieved from www.who.int/healthy_settings/en (accessed 23 January 2018).

Whitehead, M. (1991) The Concepts and Principles of Equity and Health, *Health Promotion International*, 6(3): 217–228.

Zhou, Q., Eisenberg, N., Losoya, S., Fabes, R., Reiser, M., Guthrie, I., Murphy, B. C., Cumberland, A. and Shepard, S. (2002) The Relations of Parental Warmth and Positive Expressiveness to Children's Empathy-Related Responding and Social Functioning: A Longitudinal Study, *Child Development*, 73: 893–915.

# 7

# FINDING PLAYFULNESS IN THE EVERYDAY

## An antidote to the 'saturation' of modern family life

*Julia Whitaker*

## Introduction

Families who spend time together – eating, learning, playing, and interacting with the wider community – create the strong emotional bonds and positive behaviors essential for social and emotional resilience throughout the life-cycle (Walsh 2016). This chapter explores the realities of family life in the 21st century and the implications for family cohesion and wellbeing. The rediscovery of playfulness in the context of family life is discussed in terms of the possibilities it offers for a happier and healthier lived experience of 'family', regardless of socio-economic circumstance or individual characteristics (Inspiring Scotland n.d.). Research now shows that increased opportunities for play – especially active outdoor play – contribute to physical, psychological, social and emotional development, with positive implications for reducing the influence of socio-economic differentials (ibid.).

Across the developed world, family life has undergone unprecedented change over the last 50 years. The rise in female employment has been matched by the increased educational attainment of women with a consequent postponement of parenthood, reduced family size, and a preponderance of smaller households. Fewer marriages, coupled with rising divorce rates, have contributed to an increase in one-parent families and 'blended' family arrangements. Social and geographical mobility, and the opportunities presented by the global marketplace, mean that many young families now live at a geographical distance from their kinship group, increasing the risk of social and cultural isolation. While histori-cally, the average family income has increased, there remains a significant gender gap in employment and earning potential. The United Nations Children Fund (UNICEF 2017) reports that an average of one in five children in developed nations currently live in relative poverty. More than half of UK parents believe that family life is harder now than it was two decades ago (YouGov 2014) – a perception mirrored in the US, where modern parents are found to be stressed, tired, rushed, and short on quality time (Pew Research Center 2015).

## Families saturated by choice

The relative freedoms enjoyed by the modern family – freedom from rigidly defined roles, from domestic drudgery and from economic dependence – have vastly increased the choices available to parents and children, with paradoxical consequences for family life. Schwartz (2016: 103) explains: 'Freedom and autonomy are critical to our wellbeing, and choice is critical to freedom and autonomy. Nonetheless, though modern Americans have more choice than any group of people ever has had before, and thus, presumably, more freedom and autonomy, we don't seem to be benefiting from it psychologically.' As traditional family values and systems come up against the pluralism associated with the communications revolution, the ensuing 'overchoice' (Toffler 1999) has prompted a new wave of social and psychological instability and insecurity – with serious consequences for the emotional wellbeing of the family as a unit. The family home has opened its doors to the anonymous intimacy of electronic interaction and can no longer claim to be the protected and protective refuge it once was, while the concept of a shared family narrative is challenged by a seemingly infinite array of alternative and often conflicting opinions, beliefs, and values. Gergen (1991) is credited with naming the 'saturation' of family life, which occurs when family members find themselves scattered from its core in an endless cycle of futile 'busyness'.

Gergen's appraisal of the turmoil that is modern family life is reinforced by contemporary data. The Modern Families Index 2017 reports that almost half of all couple families in the UK comprise two parents who work full-time outside the home, while 57 per cent of single parents have full-time jobs. Yet, only one in five of all parents surveyed feel that they have the right balance between time and money in order to see their family thrive (Working Families 2017). The practical challenges of modern family life, coupled with ever-increasing expectations of happiness and fulfilment (Rutledge et al. 2014), have generated the proverbial 'hamster-wheel effect' whereby many parents often feel that they are running to stand still.

## Shared obliviousness

Rosenblatt (2009) refers to the state of 'shared obliviousness' which arises from the social saturation of modern family life, narrowing the focus of attention and sapping the energy available for curiosity, empathy and re-evaluation. When the business of 'parenting' becomes just another task to be tackled, the associated worry and stress about 'getting in right' obscure the potential for a more joyful, playful experience of living as part of a family group.

Working families recognize that they are primarily responsible for finding a good work-life balance, but commonly place the onus for change elsewhere – on employers or on the state (Working Families 2017) – negating their own potential and responsibility for creating the changes they seek. Perera (2016) explains that when responsibility for change is externalized, 'we tend to focus on other people. The organisational blocks. Faults in systems. "Difficult" people who are resistant to change. Rarely do we stop to consider ourselves and the ways in which we impose limits which inhibit effective action.' Psychologist Oliver James describes this state of emotional impotence in stark terms, as 'leaving people … as much in the grip of external forces as the hypnotised or compulsively obsessed' (James 2007: 13), linking a lack of volition to the high levels of emotional distress experienced by many modern families.

The Modern Families Index (Working Families 2017) reports that only one in five families feel they have a satisfactory work-life balance. Fathers in the UK work some of the longest hours in Europe (45 hours per week) and many parents (72 per cent) do extra work at home in the evenings or at weekends. The actual or perceived need to prioritize work responsibilities has serious implications for the modern family for whom time currency is in short supply: almost half of the parents surveyed (48 per cent) for the Modern Families Index report that work gets in the way of them spending time playing and interacting with their children. The supremacy of working life is reflected in a 2016 study in the US (SWNS Digital n.d.) which found that modern families spend just thirty-eight minutes per day together, with reliance on technology disrupting available free time: 'A worrying trend to emerge is the influence our heavy reliance on electronic devices is having on the lack of quality time we spend with our loved ones, as even when we are all at home together, chances are, much of that time will be spent with children and parents staring at a screen.' (Liz Penney cited in SWNS Digital n.d.)

Parents typically agree that family is their main priority (Working Families 2017) but a focus on the world of work and all it represents (identity, status, success) inhibits consideration of other potential areas of remedial action, contributing to a 'shared obliviousness' to creative problem-solving and a collective hopelessness about the possibility of positive change.

## Health as a social movement

The public health agenda, at both national and global levels, has increasingly been shaped by recognition of the social factors influencing health and illness and the need for public, private, and community sectors to work together towards shared goals (University of Edinburgh 2017). In the UK, the National Health Service's 'Five Year Forward Review' (NHS England 2014) emphasized this shift in the power for change, from public institutions towards individuals, families and communities. Public health is increasingly recognized as a 'social movement', and people-powered lifestyle movements offer new opportunities to explore the options for health-related behavioral change at ground level (Del Castillo et al. 2016).

The call for a re-evaluation of the ways in which the global community addresses contemporary challenges to public health has never been more pressing because the health implications of a family life 'saturated' by an infinite and conflictual barrage of external demands on time and attention are significant.

- More than 1 in 2 adults and 1 in 6 children in OECD countries are overweight or obese (OECD 2017).
- In the UK, 58% of women and 68% of men are overweight or obese (NHS Digital 2017).
- 1 in 5 UK children aged 5, and 1 in 3 UK children aged 10, are overweight or obese (NHS Digital 2017).
- Just 26% of UK adults eat the recommended 5 portions of fruit and vegetables a day (NHS Digital 2017).
- 26% of UK adults take less than 30 minutes of exercise per day (NHS Digital 2017).
- It is estimated that 1 in 6 people experience a common mental health problem (Mental Health Foundation 2017).
- Major depression is thought to be the second leading cause of disability worldwide and is a major contributor to the incidence of suicide and ischemic heart disease (Mental Health Foundation 2017).
- Approximately 68% of women and 57% of men with mental health problems are parents (Mental Health Foundation 2017).

Almost half of the parents surveyed for the Modern Families Index 2017 (Working Families 2017) report that their work pattern prevents them from taking physical exercise (49 per cent) and leaves them with insufficient time to ensure a healthy diet (43 per cent). The stress associated with trying to maintain a satisfactory work-family balance negatively impacts on performance at work, creating a negative feedback loop between work and home (Burnett et al. 2012). Parents commonly report feeling 'burned-out' by the conflicting demands of work and family life (Working Families 2017) but identify change to the working aspect of their lives (taking annual/sick leave, reducing working hours, or quitting work altogether) as offering the only possibility of respite. However, there is evidence that simple, playful changes on the home-front can restore a sense of agency with a consequent impact on quality of life.

## Family cohesion, wellbeing and play

Family cohesion has been defined as 'the emotional bonding members have with one another and the degree of individual autonomy a person experiences in the family system' (Olson et al. 1979: 5). There is a well-established body of evidence for the significance of family cohesion in terms of the health and wellbeing of society (Bruhn 2009). A sense of belonging – to a family and to the wider community – serves a protective function in term of mental health (Huppert 2008), especially where family relationships are characterized by an attitude of acceptance and co-operation.

Regardless of family structure or socio-economic circumstance, one of the factors with the greatest influence on child wellbeing is the child's perception of their relationship with their parents (McKeown et al. 2003). Having a trusting, stable and supportive relationship with a parent (or parental figure) is emerging in the international literature as one of the most important aspects of childhood resilience (Bellis et al. 2017). A high level of family connection also offers physiological payback, including increased immunity to infection, a reduced risk of heart disease and delayed cognitive decline in old age (Yaxley et al. 2012).

Stinnett and DeFrain (1985) found that a key characteristic of connected, cohesive, families was that they took part in fun or playful activities together. Play energizes and creates common ground, while offering parents new perspectives through sharing a child's perception of the world (Carlson and Dermer 2016). Whether eating, cooking, gardening or just 'hanging-out' together, parents who nurture a playful attitude to life, create a 'temporary exit from normal reality' (James 2007: 423) and its inevitable demands and frustrations.

It is no coincidence that the nations at the top of happiness and wellbeing league tables – the countries in the Scandinavian triangle, Switzerland, Netherlands and Canada – are those with strong traditions of family connection through shared recreational activities (Helliwell et al. 2017). The Danes lay claim to the title of 'the happiest people in the world' and, in *The Danish Way of Parenting*, Alexander and Sandahl (2016) highlight the playfulness integral to Danish family life. The Danish concept of *hygge*, or cosiness, has found global resonance in the shared experience of emotional wellbeing when enjoying the company of family and friends: sharing meals and playing games in a spirit of intimate conviviality or togetherness (Wiking 2016). Research suggests a biological basis to the experience of *hygge* in the release of the hormone oxytocin, which is known to accompany positive physical proximity to another person and which increases subjective perceptions of wellbeing and social connection (Kosfeld et al. 2005). Playful togetherness fosters the trust and understanding essential for family cohesion and the wellbeing it engenders.

## Getting physical

Observations of the play of young children reveal that, like that of all young mammals, it is a lively, active process (Trawick-Smith 2014). A standout feature of the way in which families play together in the Nordic nations (when they are not enjoying *hyggeligt* time indoors) is that they enjoy the active, physical aspects of a playful lifestyle such as walking, cycling and spending time in nature. Family play which incorporates physical activity serves the dual benefits of nurturing filial connections while boosting exercise levels (Biddle and Ekkekakis 2005). The release of endorphins during physical activity improves mood and can transform the family dynamic, fostering a positive attitude towards exercise and physicality with lifelong benefits (Cox 2017). Children's motivation towards physical activity is both an innate disposition and an acquired attribute (Chen 2015): active play in childhood translates to healthful physical literacy throughout the life-cycle (Sport Wales 2014).

Cycling (or walking) to school or work is second nature to the Danes, 90 per cent of whom own a bicycle and who benefit from national investment in a host of cycle-friendly initiatives. The health benefits of such an active lifestyle are irrefutable: Denmark ranks 107th on the international obesity tables, despite high rates of smoking, drinking and sugar consumption (Renew Bariatrics 2017). A 2017 study reported in the *British Medical Journal* found that, as well as reducing obesity rates, cycling to work is associated with a 41 per cent lower risk of premature death, a 45 per cent lower risk of cancer and a 46 per cent lower risk of heart disease (Celis-Morales et al. 2017). Cycling and walking are natural mood-boosters (Martin et al. 2014) and offer extended opportunities for families to spend time together with a common purpose. A family ramble or cycle incorporates all the elements necessary for family connectedness: acceptance, cooperation, sharing, and playful interaction.

In the UK, the 'Big City Ride' (British Cycling 2017) is an example of a family-friendly enterprise designed to encourage families to have fun through physical activity. By opening-up the streets of some of the UK's biggest cities to bikes, the project aims to inspire families to make cycling part of their everyday lives (as it is for the Danes) with all the societal, ecological and health benefits that offers. 'Parents in Sport Week' is a parallel initiative which recognizes the pivotal role of parents in encouraging and supporting children to have a playful attitude towards sport and exercise (NSPCC 2017).

On the other side of the world in Colombia, Bogotá is one of the world's great biking cities with 350 kilometres of cycleways. Every Sunday, over 100 kilometres of the city's roads are closed to motor traffic as the city is transformed into a huge inter-generational playground. Cyclists, joggers, and skateboarders take to the streets, while the parks are occupied by free dance and exercise classes – all in a spirit of playfulness and social blending. The *Ciclovía* or 'open streets' concept has spread worldwide since its modest inception in the 1970s, with playful pursuits regularly given priority over motor traffic throughout South America and the US, and in countries as diverse as India, Israel and New Zealand (Bain 2013).

Walking and cycling are cited as examples of inexpensive activities which may be enjoyed in a spirit of playfulness by all members of the family (NHS Choices n. d.), but informal, spontaneous games such as hide-and-seek or roughhousing offer equivalent opportunities for a physical workout. Cohen (2008: 94) advocates thoughtful, physical play for all families, as a way of creating 'closeness, confidence and healing from hurts' as well as for helping children to explore and develop their physical capacities.

## Please do play at the table!

A vast body of research has found that the simple act of coming together for a family meal has a profound effect on family cohesion (e.g. Ermish et al. 2011). Family dinner is an opportunity for families to re-connect and to create a designated time and space to come together, separate from the often overwhelming demands of daily life. It may also serve as the locus for playful experimentation 'with new roles, behaviors, and patterns of communication' (Fishel 2016: 514) and, as such, is crucial to the formation of family identity.

Eating together as a family, at least once or twice a week, has been shown to have a positive influence on wellbeing, particularly on the mental health and educational attainment of children (Eisenberg et al. 2004). Strengthening family cohesion also has a positive role in promoting the physical and mental health of adolescents (Franco et al. 2008), and family connectedness, positive family communication, parental supervision, and maternal presence at mealtimes are known to protect against the onset of disordered eating patterns (Fonseca et al. 2004).

There is a significant evidence-base for the association between nutrition and physical health (Hall et al. 2011) but also robust data for the relevance of nutrition to subjective wellbeing (Sacker 2012). These benefits to health and wellbeing are further enhanced when family members – or groups of families – grow, shop or cook for meals together (Gallup et al. 2003), combining the positive aspects of physical exercise, engagement with nature, social interaction and the potential for fun! The holistic health benefits for families of sharing in the growing, preparing and eating of food is as much to do with the emotional investment in the component processes as with any nutritional gains (Story and Neumark-Sztainer 2005). Family meals include both of the elements required for family cohesion – emotional bonding through shared experience, and personal differentiation through individual contributions to the preparation and celebration of the meal. They present opportunities for parents and children to talk and laugh together, sharing the playful banter that fosters a sense of cultural identity and belonging (Office for National Statistics 2014). Sharing amusing stories and anecdotes, jokes, and wordplay creates a playful mood, builds shared memories and unifies generations.

Co-housing communities, modelled on the *bofaellesskab* which originated in Denmark (Graae 1967), are a contemporary example of neighborhood developments which exemplify the pivotal role of shared meals in creating the conditions for playful interaction and family cohesion. A central feature of the *bofaellesskab* is the large, communal kitchen and dining area where families come together to prepare meals, to eat and to socialize. When they are not part of the kitchen crew, parents are free to relax and play with their children and with neighbors. A shared vegetable garden means that families act together to grow their own fresh produce in an atmosphere which combines the work and play of family life, with positive implications for both food choices and family relations.

Since the turn of the 21st century, co-housing projects have arisen in the UK, US, Australia, New-Zealand, Canada, and Japan and it has been estimated that there exist more than 1000 functional cohousing communities, with the same number under development (Lietaert 2010). A report by the London School of Economics identifies increased physical and social resilience as one of the benefits of cohousing, resulting from improvements in living standards and 'increased self-awareness, compassionate caring and shared community knowledge' (Jarvis et al. 2016: 9). Families that live, work and play together, reap multiple benefits at individual, family and group levels.

The co-housing phenomenon is undeniably reflective of the ways in which families have traditionally connected around the globe. The proverbial concept that 'it takes a village to raise a child' predominates traditional African culture and conveys a worldview which emphasizes the value of family relationships, parental care, altruism, sharing, and hospitality (Healey and Sybertz 1997). The playfulness necessary for family cohesion, and consequently for family wellbeing, pervades many traditional cultures in which all generations live, work and play in close proximity. In Okinawa, Japan, the tradition of *moai* – the creation of informal social networks whose members commit themselves to each other for life – is another example of a lifestyle model which incorporates elements of play and playfulness. Families who belong to a *moai* are found to be happier, healthier, to experience less stress, and to live longer because their emotional, social and practical needs are entwined (Buettner 2010).

## Cultivating the family garden

The communal garden of the *bofaellesskab* serves as both an economic and a cross-generational recreational resource. Gardening for recreation and relaxation offers many of the health benefits of play in that it incorporates aspects of physical, cognitive, social and emotional life. Gardening demands an interruption of the busyness or monotony of family life, while providing an opportunity for families to re-channel physical and mental energy and to release pent-up emotions. Family-based nature activities can serve as a pathway for positive family functioning even more effectively than other types of leisure contexts (Izenstark and Ebata 2016). Having something to look forward to is a key measure of wellbeing (van Boven and Ashworth 2007) and gardening cultivates a sense of anticipation which can be shared by all members of the family (Schmutz et al. 2014).

Research suggests that the positive benefits of horticulture, for both physical and mental health, derive from the combined effects of physical activity and the consumption of fresh produce (Sommerfeld et al. 2010). Therapeutic horticulture projects improve the lives of people with a range of support needs, deploying the physical, cognitive, social and emotional aspects of gardening to enhance the lived experience of participants (Sempik et al. 2002). In Singapore, the Government has invested in healing gardens and therapeutic horticulture as a way of creating cross-generational opportunities for promoting and restoring aspects of health through engagement with a diversity of pleasurable pursuits (National Parks Board 2017).

Aside from the holistic benefits of horticulture and growing food for the family, gardening offers an apt metaphor for family life. The saturated family, overwhelmed by choice and by external demands and expectations, resembles a garden overrun with weeds. Stress and negativity can obscure the possibilities for playfulness and joy which exist to be nurtured and cultivated. The patience, perseverance and adaptability required of the gardener, reflect the pattern of repetition and variation in play, which offers the modern family an alternative to the busy monotony of an outcome-driven life. In her acclaimed book *The Gardener and the Carpenter*, developmental psychologist

Alison Gopnik draws on the gardening metaphor to advocate for a different model of family life, one in which there is interplay between the adults and children and where playfulness has the space to flourish (Gopnik 2016).

## Conclusion

Becoming a playful family 'means having an attitude that anything can be fun' (Cohen 2008: 181). Finding playfulness in the everyday does not necessarily mean finding time for a game of Ludo or looking-out the juggling balls (although those can be fun too!): going for a family ramble or bike-ride, exchanging banter round the dinner table, or growing something together, all offer opportunities for play and playfulness in the course of everyday family life – with knock-on benefits for everyone's health and wellbeing (Coyl-Shepherd and Hanlon 2013).

Governments and public institutions can facilitate family cohesion through family-friendly policies and initiatives, but the seeds of change and growth lie in the playful heart of each of us. The play drive is innate, so playfulness is not so much a skill to be learned as a gift to be re-discovered. Play is about finding alternatives, generating variability (De Koven 2014), in what we do and how we live. For the modern family, struggling to achieve a satisfactory work-life balance, finding opportunities for playfulness in everyday life can make the difference between social and emotional 'saturation' and a life worth living.

## References

Alexander, J. and Sandahl, I. (2016) *The Danish Way of Parenting*, London: Penguin.

Bain, A. (2013) Reclaiming the Streets in Bogota, retrieved from www.bbc.com/travel/story/20130828-reclaiming-the-streets-in-bogata (accessed 26 October 2017).

Bellis, M., HardcastleK., Ford, K., Hughes, K., AshtonK., Quigg, Z. and Butler, N. (2017) Does Continuous Trusted Adult Support in Childhood Impart Life-Course Resilience against Adverse Childhood Experiences – a Retrospective Study on Adult Health-Harming behaviours and Mental Well-Being, *BMC Psychiatry*, 17: 110.

Biddle, J. and Ekkekakis, P. (2005) Physically Active Lifestyles and Wellbeing, in F. Huppert, N. Baylis and B. Keveme (eds), *The Science of Well-being*, 141–170, Oxford: Oxford University Press.

British Cycling (2017) Let's Ride, retrieved from www.letsride.co.uk/city-ride (accessed 26 October 2017).

Bruhn, J. (2009) *The Group Effect: Social Cohesion and Health Outcomes*, Berlin: Springer Science and Business Media.

Buettner, D. (2010) *The Blue Zones: Lessons for Living Longer from the People Who've Lived the Longest*, Washington, DC: National Geographic.

Burnett, S., Coleman, L., Houlston, C. and Reynolds, J. (2012) *Happy Homes and Productive Workplaces. Report of Research Findings*, London: OnePlusOne.

Carlson, J. and Dermer, S. (2016) *The SAGE Encyclopedia of Marriage, Family, and Couples Counseling*, Thousand Oaks, CA: Sage Publications.

Celis-Morales, C., Lyall, D., Welsh, P., AndersonJ., SteellL., GuoY., Maldonado, R., Mackay, D., Pell, J.Sattar, N. and Gill, J. (2017) Association between Active Commuting and Incident Cardiovascular Disease, Cancer, and Mortality: Prospective Cohort Study, *British Medical Journal*, 357: j1456.

Chen, A. (2015) Operationalizing Physical Literacy for Learners: Embodying the Motivation to Move, *Journal of Sport and Health Science*, 4(2): 125–131.

Cohen, L. (2008) *Playful Parenting: An Exciting New Approach to Raising Children That Will Help You Nurture Close Connections, Solve Behavior Problems, and Encourage Confidence*, New York: Random House.

Cox, D. (2017) Young at Heart: Why Children Who Exercise Become Healthier Adults, retrieved from www.theguardian.com/lifeandstyle/2017/aug/28/young-at-heart-why-children-who-exercise-become-healthier-adults (accessed 2 May 2018).

Coyl-Shepherd, D. and Hanlon, C. (2013) Family Play and Leisure Activities: Correlates of Parents' and Children's Socio-emotional Well-being, *International Journal of Play*, 2(3): 254–272.

De Koven, B. (2014) *A Playful Path*, North Carolina: Lulu.com.

Del Castillo, J., Khan, H., Nicholas, L. and Finnis, A. (2016) *Health as a Social Movement. The Power of People in Movements*, London: Nesta.

Eisenberg, M., Olson, R., Neumark-Sztainer, D., Story, M. and BearingerL. (2004) Correlations between Family Meals and Psychosocial Well-being among Adolescents, *Archives of Pediatrics and Adolescent Medicine*, 158: 792–796.

Ermish, J., Iacovou, M. and Skew, A. (2011) Family relationships, in S. McFall, and C. Garrington (eds), *Understanding Society: Early Findings from the First Wave of the UK's Household Longitudinal Study*, 7–14, Colchester: Institute for Social and Economic Research, University of Essex.

Fishel, A. (2016) Harnessing the Power of Family Dinners to Create Change in Family Therapy, *Australia and New Zealand Journal of Family Therapy*, 37: 514–527.

Fonseca, H., Ireland, M. and Resnick, M. (2004) Familial Correlates of Extreme Weight Control Behaviors among Adolescents, *International Journal of Eating Disorders*, 32: 441–448.

Franco, D., Thompson, D., Bauserman, R. and Striegel Weissman, R. (2008) What's Love Got to Do with It? Family Cohesion and Healthy Eating Behaviors in Adolescent Girls, *International Journal of Eating Disorders*, 41: 360–367.

Gallup, S., Syracuse, C.and Oliveri, M. (2003) *What the Research Tells Us About Family Meals*, Columbus, OH: Family and Consumer Sciences, Ohio State University Extension.

Gergen, K. J. (1991) *The Saturated Self: Dilemmas of Identity in Contemporary Life*, New York: HarperCollins.

Gopnik, A. (2016) *The Gardener and the Carpenter: What the New Science of Child Development Tells Us about the Relationship Between Parents and Children*, New York: Farrar Straus and Giroux.

Graae, B. (1967) *Børn skal have Hundrede Foraeldre* [*Children Should Have One Hundred Parents*], Copenhagen: Politiken.

HallJ., d'Ardenne, J., Barnes, M., Roberts, C. and McManusS. (2011) *Food Choices and behaviour: Trends and the Impact of Life Events*, London: NatCen.

Healey, J. and Sybertz, D. (1997) *Towards an African Narrative Theology*, New York: Orbis Books.

Helliwell, J., Layard, R. and Sachs, J. (2017) *World Happiness Report 2017*, New York: Sustainable Development Solutions Network.

Huppert F. (2008) *Psychological Well-being: Evidence Regarding its Causes and its Consequences*, London: Foresight Mental Capital and Wellbeing Project BIS.

Inspiring Scotland (n.d.) Raising Attainment through Active Play, retrieved from www.insp iringscotland.org.uk/wp-content/uploads/2017/04/Active-Play-Attainment-Prospectus-F INAL.pdf (accessed 2 May 2018).

Izenstark, D. and Ebata, A. T. (2016) Theorizing Family-Based Nature Activities and Family Functioning: The Integration of Attention Restoration Theory with a Family Routines and Rituals Perspective, *Journal of Family Theory and Review*, 8: 137–153.

James, O. (2007) *Affluenza*, London: Vermillion.

Jarvis, H., Scanlon, K. and Fernández Arrigoitia, M. (2016) Cohousing: Shared Futures, retrieved from www.lse.ac.uk/geography-and-environment/assets/Documents/LSE-London/Rep orts/Cohousing-shared-futures-FINAL-web.pdf?from_serp=1 (accessed 3 October 2017).

Kosfeld, M., Heinrichs, M., Zak, P. J., Fischbacher, U. and Feh, E. (2005) Oxytocin Increases Trust in Humans, *Nature*, 435: 673–676.

Lietaert, M. (2010) Cohousing's Relevance to Degrowth Theories, *Journal of Cleaner Production*, 18: 576–580.

McKeown, K., Pratschke J. and Haase T. (2003) *Family Wellbeing: What Makes a Difference; Study Based on a Representative Sample of Parents and Children in Ireland*, Shannon, Ireland: The Céifin Centre.

Martin, A., Goryakin, Y. and Suhrcke, M. (2014) Does Active Commuting Improve Psychological Wellbeing? Longitudinal Evidence from Eighteen Waves of the British Household Panel Survey, *Preventive Medicine*, 69: 296–303.

Mental Health Foundation (2017) Mental Health Statistics: UK and Worldwide, retrieved from www.mentalhealth.org.uk/statistics/mental-health-statistics-uk-and-worldwide (accessed 9 October 2017).

National Parks Board (2017) Therapeutic Gardens, retrieved from www.nparks.gov.sg/ga rdens-parks-and-nature/therapeutic-gardens (accessed 3 October 2017).

NHS Choices (n.d.) Get Fit for Free, retrieved from www.nhs.uk/Livewell/fitness/Pages/ free-fitness.aspx (accessed 25 October 2017).

NHS Digital (2017) Statistics on Obesity, Physical Activity and Diet. England: 2017, retrieved from www.gov.uk/government/uploads/system/uploads/attachment_data/file/ 613532/obes-phys-acti-diet-eng-2017-rep.pdf (accessed 9 October 2017).

NHS England (2014) Five Year Forward View, retrieved from www.england.nhs.uk/wp -content/uploads/2014/10/5yfv-web.pdf (accessed 9 October 2017).

NSPCC (2017) Parents in Sport, retrieved from https://thecpsu.org.uk/help-advice/top ics/parents-in-sport (accessed 26 October 2017).

OECD (2017) Obesity Update 2017, retrieved from www.oecd.org/els/health-systems/ Obesity-Update-2017.pdf (accessed 9 October 2017).

Office for National Statistics (2014) Measuring National Well-being: Children's Well-being, retrieved from http://webarchive.nationalarchives.gov.uk/20160107224139/www.ons. gov.uk/ons/dcp171776_355140.pdf (accessed 9 October 2017).

Olson, D., Sprenkle, D. and Russell, C. (1979) Circumplex Model of Marital and Family Systems: I. Cohesion and Adaptability Dimension, Family Types and Applications, *Family Process*, 18, 3–28.

Perera, K. (2016) 3 Tips for Creating a Social Movement, retrieved from www.thersa.org/ discover/publications-and-articles/rsa-blogs/2016/09/3-tips-for-creating-a-social-movem ent (accessed 9 October 2017).

Pew Research Center (2015) Raising Kids and Running a Household: How Working Parents Share the Load, retrieved from www.pewsocialtrends.org/2015/11/04/raising-kids-and-run ning-a-household-how-working-parents-share-the-load (accessed 12 October 2017).

Renew Bariatrics (2017) Report: Obesity Rates by Country – 2017, retrieved from https:// renewbariatrics.com/obesity-rank-by-countries (accessed 26 October 2017).

Rosenblatt, P. (2009) *Shared Obliviousness in Family Systems*, New York: Suny Press.

Rutledge, R., Skandali, N., Dayan, P. and Dolan, R. (2014) A Computational and Neural Model of Momentary Subjective Wellbeing, *Proceedings of the National Academy of Sciences USA*, 111(33): 12, 252–212, 257.

SWNS Digital (n.d.) Families Spend Less than 40 Minutes a Day Together, retrieved from www.swnsdigital.com/2016/03/families-spend-less-than-40-minutes-a-day-together (accessed 03 October 2017).

Sacker, A. (2012) Health Related behaviours and Wellbeing in Adolescence, retrieved from www.ucl.ac.uk/iehc/research/epidemiology-public-health/research/international-cen tre-for-lifecourse-studies/publications/op/op9_2.pdf (accessed 7 September 2018).

Schmutz, U., Lennartsson, M., Williams, S., Devereaux, M. and Davies, G. (2014) *The Benefits of Gardening and Food Growing for Health and Wellbeing*, London: Garden Organic and Sustain.

Schwartz, B. (2016) *The Paradox of Choice: Why More is Less. How the Culture of Abundance Robs Us of Satisfaction*, New York: HarperCollins.

Sempik, J., Aldridge, J. and Becke, S. (2002) *Social and Therapeutic Horticulture: Evidence and Messages from Research*, Reading: Thrive (in association with the Centre for Child and Family Research).

Sommerfeld, A., Mcfarland, A., Waliczek, T. and ZajicekJ. (2010) Growing Minds: Evaluating the Relationship between Gardening and Fruit and Vegetable Consumption in Older Adults, *Hort Technology*, 20: 711–717.

Sport Wales (2014) Physical Literacy. A Journey through Life, retrieved from http://physica lliteracy.sportwales.org.uk/en (accessed 3 May 2018).

Stinnett, N. and DeFrain, J. (1985) *Secrets of Strong Families*, Boston, MA: Little Brown.

Story, M., and Neumark-Sztainer, D. (2005) A Perspective on Family Meals: Do They Matter?, *Nutrition Today*, 40(6): 261–266.

Toffler, A. (1999) *Future Shock*, St Louis, MO: Turtleback Books.

Trawick-Smith, J. (2014) The Physical Play and Motor Development of Young Children: A Review of Literature and Implications for Practice, retrieved from www.easternct.edu/ cece/files/2014/06/BenefitsOfPlay_LitReview.pdf (accessed 26 October 2017).

UNICEF (2017) *Building the Future: Children and the Sustainable Development Goals in Rich Countries*, Florence: UNICEF Office of Research – Innocenti.

University of Edinburgh (2017) Social Determinants of Health and Public Policy, retrieved from www.socialpolicy.ed.ac.uk/research/research_groups/global_public_health_unit/ social_determinants_of_health_and_public_policy (accessed 9 October 2017).

Van Boven, L. and Ashworth, L. (2007) Looking Forward, Looking Back: Anticipation Is More Evocative Than Retrospection, *Journal of Experimental Psychology*, 136(2): 289–300.

Walsh, F. (2016) Family Resilience: A Developmental Systems Framework, *European Journal of Developmental Psychology*, 13(3), retrieved from http://dx.doi.org/10.1080/17405629. 2016.1154035 (accessed 7 September 2018).

Wiking, M. (2016) *The Little Book of Hygge*, London: Penguin.

Working Families (2017) The Modern Families Index, retrieved from www.workingfam ilies.org.uk/wp-content/uploads/2017/01/Modern-Families-Index_Full-Report.pdf (accessed 22 September 2017).

Yaxley, V., Gill, V. and McManus, S. (2012) *Family Wellbeing: Measuring What Matters*, London: NatCen Social Research.

YouGov (2014) Over Half of Parents Believe Family Life is Harder than it Was Twenty Years Ago, retrieved from https://yougov.co.uk/news/2014/01/15/over-half-parents-be lieve-family-life-harder-it-wa (accessed 12 October 2017).

# 8

# THE PLAYFUL PURSUIT OF CHILD PUBLIC HEALTH

*Jenni Etchells and Alison Tonkin*

## Introduction

Children and adolescents make up over 20 per cent of the global population and healthy, happy children are likely to become healthy, happy and productive adults (Blair et al. 2010). Child public health plays a major role in promoting holistic health and wellbeing, not just for children and adolescents themselves, but also for their families and local communities within the broader social and political land-scapes (ibid.). Public health is a multifaceted and intricate 'art' which focuses not just on the eradication of disease but on the complete spectrum of health and wellbeing (World Health Organization 2018a). The World Health Organization (2018b) has a key role in providing leadership, shaping the research agenda and monitoring health trends across the globe, while national governments are required to adopt 'whole society' and 'whole government' approaches to public health that represent the societies they serve (World Health Organization 2012).

This chapter will explore how play and playfulness contribute to the public health agenda for children and adolescents, acknowledging the central role of play in helping children to reach their full potential (APPG on a Fit and Healthy Childhood 2015). According to the All Party Parliamentary Group on a Fit and Healthy Childhood (ibid.), today's children, named Generation Z, need play to promote physical activity as well as to enhance development in the areas of cognitive, emotional, social and nutritional health. There are calls for public health to 'learn from the evidence and give play its place within the strategies and initiatives that they devise with the aim of creating a world in which Generation Z and their successors can feel at home and flourish' (ibid.: 53). However, there are risks to 'utilizing' play as a means of achieving public health outcomes. These include, for example, using play as a tool to reduce obesity or to increase physical activity – as opposed to promoting play for play's sake (Alexander 2011). *Active play* is defined as unstructured physical activity which typically takes place in a child's free time, following their own agenda in an outdoor environment (Brockman et al. 2011). Increasing physical activity through structured, adult-led interventions potentially misses the unique contribution of child-led *active play* which, in addition to promoting physical health, also enhances creativity and offers opportunities for informal social engagement, conflict resolution and enjoyment (ibid.). This chapter focuses on the self-reinforcing pleasure that play brings through reward pathways in the brain (Perry et al. 2000), exploring play-based strategies that are rooted in the edutainment and playful engagement of children and adolescents.

## Exploring child and adolescent health and development

Between 2015 and 2018, the World Bank Group (2018) published, under the third edition of the Disease Control Priorities (*DCP3*) series, nine volumes linked to efforts to quantify the sustainable development goal for health (SDG). This chapter has used *Volume 8 – Child and Adolescent Health and Development* (World Bank Group 2018) as the platform for exploring key themes linked to public health for children and adolescents. Although play is rarely mentioned, it is evident that the processes of play and playful engagement have been adapted, through differentiation, to develop interventions that are both effective and fun for the target audience (Tonkin and Weldon 2013).

The former British prime minister Gordon Brown (cited in World Bank Group 2018: xiv) wrote the Foreword for *Volume 8*, emphasizing one of its key messages, namely that 'human development is a slow process: it takes two decades – 8,000 days – for a human to develop physically and mentally'. Recognizing the intertwined nature of health, nutrition and education from the age of 5 to 19 years of age, the World Group Bank (ibid.) identify the lifelong consequences of this whole formative period. These had previously been noted by Zimmerman and Woolf (2014) who articulated that health is a foundation for learning, while education is a determinant of health.

Bundy et al. (2017: 1) suggest that, 'research and action on child health and development should evolve from the narrow emphasis of the first 1,000 days to holistic concern over the first 8,000 days; from an age-siloed approach to an approach that embraces the needs across the life cycle' as demonstrated in Table 8.1.

Bundy and Horton (2017) identify that each developmental stage is critical for supporting subsequent development and for reinforcing the achievements made during earlier stages. As the child progresses through these stages, into adolescence and finally adulthood, the health-related themes also change, although some themes will progress with the child. Bruner's (1977: 33) concept of the *spiral curriculum*, provides a framework for differentiating public health interventions by reviewing and updating information in a spiral fashion, revisiting topics on a regular basis and growing in complexity as the child progresses through the developmental stages (Tonkin 2007).

The remainder of this chapter examines four examples which demonstrate how play approaches vary according to the developmental phase under consideration.

**TABLE 8.1** Key phases of child and adolescent health and development linked to public health interventions.

| Phase | Period | Developmental importance to public health | Intervention themes |
|---|---|---|---|
| The first 1000 days | Conception to age 2 years | Most rapid period of growth and development that underpins all subsequent development. Has the highest risk of mortality. | Immunization Vaccination Mandatory |
| Preschoolers *Note: this age range is not featured as one of the four critical phases in the original table* | *Ages 3 to 4 years* | *Emergence of social skills, especially important for emerging self-esteem and learning. Physical development is more energetic and coordinated (State Government of Victoria 2017). Together with 1–2 year olds, most at risk from accidents in the home (RoSPA 2018).* | *Accident prevention Physical activity Oral health and hygiene Social and emotional behavior* |
| Middle childhood (growth and consolidation) | Ages 5 to 9 years | Steady physical growth with development of sensorimotor functionality of the brain. Infection and malnutrition are key constraints on development. | Infection control Promotion of healthy behaviors and wellbeing Diet and nutrition |
| Adolescent growth spurt | Ages 10 to 14 years | Rapid growth in physical and emotional centers of development. 'Significant physiological and behavioral changes associated with puberty' (Bundy and Horton 2017: 2). | 'Age appropriate variations on the above' Vaccination Physical activity Promotion of healthy emotional development |
| Adolescent growth and consolidation | Ages 15 to 19 years | Consolidation of physical growth and brain restructuring; risk-taking behavior linked with 'exploration and experimentation and initiation of behaviors that are life-long determinants of health' (Bundy and Horton 2017: 2). | Reproductive health Incentives to stay in school Protection from excessive risk taking Early identification of mental health issues |

Source: adapted from Bundy and Horton (2017)

## Promotion – oral health and hygiene

Oral diseases are one of the most common type of diseases worldwide, with tooth decay representing the highest global burden, affecting 3.1 billion people (Benzian et al. 2017). In June 2017, Public Health England reiterated that tooth decay, which is largely preventable, is a serious problem for children and adolescents (White 2017), a situation reflected throughout the world (Benzian et al. 2017).

In the United Kingdom, it is believed that 3.3 million young people aged 0–14 years of age have already developed tooth decay (Oral Health Foundation 2016). Aside from the financial implications of healthcare interventions linked to poor oral hygiene, and the loss of school days for children and working days for parents (White 2017), tooth decay results in unnecessary pain and distress for children. White (ibid.) found that 67 per cent of parents report that their child experiences pain because of tooth decay and 38 per cent report that their child suffers sleepless nights as a result of this pain, demonstrating that poor dental health impacts on the holistic health and wellbeing, not only of the child, but also of the whole family.

Using a playful approach to encourage children to practice good oral hygiene is not a recent phenomenon. In 1983, *Practical dental health education: A guide to home-made resources and ideas* was written by Wilson (1983) and still represents the foundation of the oral health practices we teach our children today. It featured adaptations of children's games such as Snakes and Ladders to promote good oral health and hygiene and the game can still be downloaded from the British Dental Association (2018) website.

There is an understanding that a child's early experience of oral health can impact on them for the rest of their lives (Oral Health Foundation 2016) and that resources which integrate public health messages into everyday play experiences are very effective. Preparing children for their first visit to the dentist should start at an early age, involving children through focused discussion, using fictional characters that children can engage with (Crystal 2010).

Monkey Wellbeing has produced an activity pack (Figure 8.1) to promote oral health which includes a storybook (*Monkey's Family Visits the Dentist*) and an activity guide (*Monkey's Guide to Healthy Teeth*) which have been written in collaboration with practicing dental health practitioners and with advice and support from the British Dental Health Foundation. The pack includes stickers, colored pencils, a laminated teeth-cleaning chart with dry-wipe pen, and a certificate (Monkey Wellbeing 2018). The *Monkey* publications provide a fun and entertaining way to generate discussion, presenting a mixture of facts, games and puzzles in a manner which appeals to children to promote their active engagement in caring for their own oral health.

*Peppa Pig Visits the Dentist* (Ladybird 2015) is another playful approach to promoting oral health. Peppa Pig is a little pig who, with her brother George, encounters many adventures with her family and friends, which include the portrayal of public health engagement. Known in over 170 countries and translated into 40 different languages (Marlow 2015), Peppa Pig has inadvertently become a valuable health promotion resource.

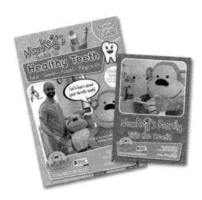

**FIGURE 8.1** Monkey wellbeing resources.
Source: reproduced by kind permission of AhHa Publications Ltd

Throughout the world, school-based interventions are a popular public health strategy. They largely focus on activities designed to develop children's skills and hygiene habits with the aim of improving their oral health (Benzian et al. 2017). Story books, DVDs, CDs and catchy songs all form part of the health-promotion toolkit, as well as daily tooth-brushing time at school as a group activity which every child can take part in and which reinforces healthy social norms (ibid.). Public health relies on population-wide interventions and, in the case of oral health policies, education, agriculture, transportation, water, sanitation and healthy nutrition all play a part in ensuring the integration of sustainable and scalable oral health interventions (ibid.).

The use of dental braces is common for children aged over seven years of age, particularly during adolescence. Braces are used to straighten crooked or protruding teeth, to close gaps between teeth and/or to correct the bite of teeth (NHS Choices 2015). Between 2014 and 2015, it was estimated that 202,300 children and young people in England and Wales started orthodontic treatment (ibid.), while in America the number is estimated at 3.3 million (Phillips 2018). The presence of braces amplifies the need for good oral hygiene, at the same time making it more challenging to achieve (Zotti et al. 2016). Many orthodontists offer children and adolescents the opportunity to have colored bands or other ornamentation on their fixed braces to introduce a personalized and fun element to the treatment, while encouraging children and young people to look after their braces and to feel more in control of their oral hygiene (Dental Associates 2018). Children and young people can personalize their braces by choosing different colors of bands to match, for example, a favourite football team, a special outfit (i.e. a family wedding) or their school uniform.

A study carried out in Italy found that employing social technologies to engage adolescents, helped to improve their compliance with oral health routines during orthodontic treatment (Zotti et al. 2016). This study asked a group of adolescents to upload weekly selfies to a WhatsApp-based chat room and found that this was done with enthusiasm and active participation, suggesting the selfie group were more compliant with an oral hygiene regime compared with a control group (ibid.).

## Prevention – respiratory health and hand hygiene

Aside from vaccination, the spread of respiratory diseases such as flu can most effectively be prevented through hygiene measures (Public Health England 2015). In 2009, the infectious disease *swine flu* (H1N1) was discovered in Mexico, triggering fears of a global pandemic (McVeigh and Tuckman 2009). In the UK, the *Catch It, Bin It, Kill It* campaign was launched in response to the spread of swine flu, urging everyone to 'carry tissues and to use them to catch coughs or sneezes, to bin the used tissues as soon as possible and then to wash their hands and kill the germs' (Phin, cited in Public Health England 2015). As well as media coverage for the general population, the campaign also had resources for different age ranges.

### *'Catch It, Bin It, Kill It'*

This rhyme, featured in Figure 8.2, targeted preschool children by using repetitive, simple lyrics and accompanying actions which could be learnt by rote and sung as part of a group activity. It is widely acknowledged that, from an early age, children are building schemas to organize their growing body of knowledge (Kumar et al. 2018). The delivery of public health strategies is a core feature of the early years curriculum, since patterns of health-related behavior established in the early years become life-long habits (Blair et al. 2010).

CATCH IT, BIN IT, KILL IT   NHS
RHYME

I will catch those germs when I "ATICHOO!",
I will catch those germs in my tissue

Catch It and Bin It to Kill It, that's it!
there're no germs on us!

Put the tissue into a bin,
germs won't get out once they are in

Catch It and Bin It to Kill It, that's it!
there're no germs on us!

Kill the germs they make us sick,
come on everyone wash them off quick!

Catch It and Bin It to Kill It, that's it!
there're no germs on us!

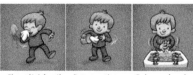

Shout 'Atichoo!'     Put your tissue     Rub your hands
and catch your       in the bin in       together quickly
sneeze or cough in   the middle of
your clean tissue    the room

**FIGURE 8.2** 'Catch it, Bin it, Kill It' poster.
Source: Department of Health (2008); Open Government Licence 2.0 (www.nationalarchives.gov.uk/doc/open-government-licence/version/2)

## Dirty Bertie – 'Catch It, Bin It, Kill It'

Dirty Bertie is a well-known character in children's literature, most popular with children between five and eleven years of age. The stories portray the 'not so nice side' of a typical little boy, with themes covering a range of unsavoury, unhygienic habits and their consequences (Book Trust 2017). The 'Catch It, Bin It, Kill It' story portrayed 'a day of hygiene horrors, with Bertie coughing and sneezing over family and friends before finally learning the right behavior thanks to expert advice from his canine companion, Whiffer' (Ohlden 2008).

The added benefit of teaching young children about good respiratory and hand hygiene is that information provided to the children can also be shared with their parents and carers. The above interventions were accompanied by printable handouts which were taken home by the children to share with their families. This is important as research undertaken by the Department of Health in 2008 revealed that 84 per cent of 1000 mothers were teaching their children the incorrect routine for dealing with coughs and sneezes (Ohlden 2008). The research also noted that 52 per cent of the mothers instructed their children to use their hands to cover their nose or mouth and none told their children to wash their hands after sneezing or coughing into their hands, meaning germs would be immediately spread to the next thing the child touched (ibid.).

## 'Swine Flu Skank'

Sawyer et al. (2017: 299) identify that 'as with all health actions, engaging young people in the development of m-health resources would help to ensure that this approach meets their needs'. As an example, CheesyBanana2009 wrote the 'Swine Flu Skank'. The verb *skank* means 'to perform a particular style of dance to ska music' (Online Slang Dictionary 2018). The artist Uproar performed the 'Swine Flu Skank' in a video which featured members of the public 'doing the skank' and this was uploaded on the social media platform YouTube (UproarUnLtd 2009).

Lyrics articulated the consistent 'Catch It, Bin It, Kill It' message as well as portraying the potentially fatal effects of swine flu:

> Do the dancePlease get with it
> (yo) …
> Catch it, Bin it, kill it etc. …
> Don't come here with your flu symptoms
> Coz I don't wanna die dude
> (yo) …
> Catch it, Bin it, kill it etc. …
>                    *(CheesyBanana2009 2009)*

JuxtaPoser (2009) commented on the effectiveness of this approach:

> The government spent some £6 million on the media awareness campaign for Swine Flu … My peeps @ Uproar come with a street video that gets 12,000+ hits in less than 24 hours. Gordon Brown should have commissioned this, instead!

## Protection – Sun safe

Encouraging children and their families to adopt a healthy lifestyle now requires consideration of environmental determinants which might counteract the benefit of an active, outdoor lifestyle. The World Health Organization (2018a) warns that a rise in the prevalence of skin cancer correlates with the increased popularity of outdoor activities and recreational exposure. Experts suggest that 80 per cent of skin cancer diagnoses could be prevented, since ultra-violet (UV) damage is largely avoidable. UV damage affects the skin, eyes and immune system (United States Environmental Protection Agency 2017) and, as children are in an active state of growth, they are more susceptible to environmental variables than adults. Most sun damage occurs due to exposure before the age of 18 years (World Health Organization 2018b). Health promotion efforts have therefore focused on school-based strategies to engage and empower children regarding sun safety.

In the United Kingdom, the Sun Safe Schools Accreditation Scheme, developed by the skin cancer charity Skcin, assists primary schools in raising awareness of the importance of sun safety and in promoting sun-safe behavior (Sun Safe Schools 2018). Various resources are available for schools, including assembly templates, lesson plans, UV monitoring resources and a rhyming, illustrated story-book entitled *George the Sunsafe Superstar*. These resources are mirrored in Australia where the national SunSmart programme has been running since 1988. Making schools a delivery platform for the encouragement of health-protection behaviors has numerous benefits, namely a captive audience and the community-wide availability of teachers to deliver simple health interventions (Department of Education and Childhood Development 2007).

Another global campaign promoting sun safety is the international bespoke sun-safety song 'Slip, Slop, Slap, Seek, Slide' which has been recognized as one of Australia's most successful health campaigns (Cancer Council Australia 2018):

> Slip on a t-shirt,
> Slop on the sunscreen,
> Slap on a hat with a wide brim,
> Seek shade between 11am and 3pm and
> Slide on your sunglasses.

Released in 1981 and updated in 2007, this song remains the preferred sun safety promotion tool around the world and has been adapted for use in pre-school, secondary school and, in New Zealand, as a short horror film targeted at adolescents and adults to drive home the sun safe message (Scoop 2017).

In the United States there is a *Sun Safe Patch* programme for the Girl Scouting movement, aimed at girls aged five to 18 years of age. To obtain the *sun safe patch* the girls must collectively complete activities based on three themes:

- Sun Savvy – activities introducing sun safety concepts.
- Sun protection – activities applying sun safe knowledge.
- Sun-Sational – activities promoting positive sun aspects.

*(Girl Scout Council of the Nation's Capital 2010)*

These activities also include an emphasis on family learning which is important because the sun protection practices of children are directly linked to the attitudes of their parents (Department of Education and Childhood Development 2007).

Games are a popular format for enhancing the protection of health and there are numerous examples of computer games available in age-appropriate formats on the internet. The aim of these bright, colorful games is to encourage engagement with recommended sun-safe behaviors. Although recognized as potentially highly effectual methods for increasing knowledge and changing behaviors, additional research is needed to ensure that the game designs enhance the effectiveness of the intended message (as noted in Chapter 9) and minimize any adverse effects that might result from the playing of computer games (Baranowski et al. 2016).

## Holistic health and wellbeing – Scouting

Scouting is 'the world's leading educational youth organization', with over 40 million active members and a mission to create a better world, according to their website (see www.scout.org). Scouting is promoted as 'education for life':

> We achieve … youth empowerment
> We create … active citizens
> We cultivate … lifelong values and skills
> We engage … in peace [and] Education.

*(www.scout.org)*

In the UK, Scouting is the biggest mixed, volunteer-led organization for young people aged six to 25 years of age, providing 'fun, challenge and adventure for more than 450,000 girls and boys' (Scout Association 2018a). With 'something for everybody', scouting provides opportunities for fun and friendship, for getting outdoors, and for the expression of creativity through a diverse range of hobbies and recreational activities, while making a positive contribution to communities by helping others (Scout Association 2018b). Each of these elements has a contribution to make to the public health agenda which exemplifies the differentiation of develop-mental stages presented in Table 8.2. For example, the need to build resilience as part of the public health agenda has been identified as a significant contributor to successful outcomes for young people (Association for Young People's Health 2016). However,

**TABLE 8.2** Scout Association section badges and awards that link to public health.

| | Cooking | Health and Fitness | Hobbies and creativity | Personal safety | Community |
|---|---|---|---|---|---|
| **Beavers** 6–8 years | Cook Healthy eating | Health & Fitness Cyclist Sports | Imagination Collector Gardener Photographer Creative Hobbies | Safety | Disability awareness Global issues |
| **Cubs** 8–10 1/2 years | Chef Backwoods Cooking | Athletics Cyclist Martial Arts Physical recreation Pioneer Skater Sports enthusiast Water activities | Animal Carer Artist Astronomer Book Reader Collector DIY Entertainer Equestrian Gardener Hobbies Photographer | Fire Safety Home Safety Personal Safety Road Safety | Disability awareness World Faiths Environmental Conservation |
| **Scouts** 10 1/2-14 years | Chef – Indoors and Outdoors | Athletics Climber Cyclist Dragon Boating Hill walker Martial Arts Physical recreation Snowsports Street Sports | Air spotter Angler Artist Circus skills Craft Farming Geocaching Hobbies Model Maker Writer | Fire safety Survival skills | Fundraiser Global issues Global faiths |
| **Explorers** 14–18 years | Challenge Chef | Challenge Athletics Climber Hillwalker Motor Sports Mountain biking Physical recreation Skiing Snowboarding Street Sports Racquet Sports | Challenge Creative arts Performing Arts | Caving Survival skills | Fundraiser Global issues Explorer belt |
| **Scout Network** 18–25 years | Take part in a range of activities that are organized and managed by themselves, including abseiling, camping, circus skills, climbing, go-karting, gorge walking, hiking, pioneering and watersports. | | | | |

'promoting resilience does not necessarily mean removing risk – it means shoring up the resources for dealing with it' (ibid.: 5). Scouting promotes age-appropriate challenge and risk-taking which reflects the interests and hobbies of young people, through the activity badges and awards that scouts can achieve as they progress through the different sections of the organization (Scout Association 2018c). A flexible approach to engagement in all aspects of the Scouting programmes means requirements for badges and awards can be adapted to ensure all young people face a 'similar level of challenge' according to their individual abilities. Table 8.2 identifies a selection of badges and challenge awards that reflect playful endeavors, including creativity and physical activities that also promote public health (although this is not the primary purpose of offering these badges and awards).

There is also a range of Staged Activity badges that progress through the sections as the young people grow and develop. These include themes such as community impact, emergency aid, hikes away, musician, paddle sports, sailing, snowsports and swimmer – a pertinent example of Bruner's Spiral Curriculum in practice.

Many scouting's badges and awards involve young people sharing their hobbies and interests with their peers and designing promotional material linked to the badge content. For example, for the Beaver Health and Fitness badge, Beavers have to 'promote healthy eating and exercise to others. This could involve designing a poster, acting out a sketch, or creating something digitally' (Scout Association 2018e). For the Explorer *Street Sports* badge, Explorers are asked to 'demonstrate skills in your chosen sport to your Unit and undertake a street sport together' (Scout Association 2018f). The evidence shows that playful, intrinsically motivated activities are much more effective in changing behavior than externally imposed initiatives (Brockman et al. 2011). As seen with the 'Swine Flu Skank', actively involving young people in developing and producing their own promotional material and resources empowers and enhances engagement with the public health message.

'Arts and creativity and are being squeezed out of schools' (BBC News 2015) and scouting's promotion of a diverse range of creative and artistic endeavors has therefore become increasingly important for young people, particularly for those from disadvantaged backgrounds. The All Party Parliamentary Group on Arts, Health and Wellbeing make the point that schools are currently failing to make the connection between health and the arts and are thus missing opportunities to promote the cultural wellbeing, mental health and holistic wellbeing of all pupils (APPG on Arts, Health and Wellbeing 2017). Research has now confirmed that, with its emphasis on fun for all age groups including the older 18–25 years age range, 'Scouting develops socially engaged young people – individuals who are curious, kind, welcoming, active, resilient and extraordinarily equipped with skills for life … [and] strengthens communities and contributes to greater social cohesion' (Scout Association 2018d).

# Conclusion

Involving children and young people as active participants in the public health agenda is an absolute necessity. Using play-based strategies such as songs, rhymes and dance as a means of engaging children and adolescents represents an element of active engagement, especially when the resources are produced by the children and adolescents themselves. This in turn empowers and enhances efficacy, since participation through informed choice is a more effective means of promoting positive health behaviors. Ensuring that children have time for play, and access to play and recreational opportunities that are fun and freely chosen, will go a long way to enabling children to build resilience and have a healthy and happy childhood. When there is a need for action to prevent illness or to protect or promote health, asking the opinions of children and young people about how they would engage their peers is crucial. They are the experts in their own communities and have much to offer to the dynamic and ever-changing world of child public health: 'We must keep engaging young people in solutions – they have creative and innovative ideas when asked ... lots of ideas' (Evans 2018).

# References

Alexander, S. (2011) Students' Den: 'All Work and No Play ... ?' A Project Investigating the Public Health Discourse on Children's Play, retrieved from http://blogs.springer.com/ijph/food-for-thought/students-den-all-work-and-no-play-a-project-investigating-the-public-health-discourse-on-childrens-play (accessed 15 March 2018).

APPG on a Fit and Healthy Childhood (2015) Play: A Report by the All Party Parliamentary Group on a Fit and Healthy Childhood, retrieved from https://mega.nz/#!9slnBDgA!WMpwXAwksLSasGpU_4oLx9I9ngnDuPjveTr_gVIFfLU (accessed 15 March 2018).

APPG on Arts, Health and Wellbeing (2017) *Creative Health: The Arts for Health and Wellbeing* [The Short Report], London: All Party Parliamentary Group on Arts, Health and Wellbeing.

Association for Young People's Health (2016) *A Public Health Approach to Promoting Young People's Resilience*, London: AYPH.

Baranowski, T., Blumberg, F., BudayR., DeSmetA., FiellinL., GreenS., Kato, P., Lu, A., Maloney, A., MelleckerR., Morrill, B., Peng, W., Shegog, R., Simons, M., Staiano, A., Thompson, D. and Young, K. (2016) Games for Health for Children – Current Status and Research Needed. *Games for Health Journal*, 5(1):1–12.

BBC News (2015) Arts and Creativity 'Squeezed Out of Schools, retrieved from www.bbc.co.uk/news/education-31518717 (accessed 17 March 2018).

Benzian, H., Garg, R., Monse, B., Staug, N. and Varenne, B. (2017) Promoting Oral Health through Programs in Middle Childhood and Adolescence, in World Bank Group, *Disease Control Priorities, Third Edition: Child and Adolescent Health and Development*, 211–220, Washington, DC: World Bank Group.

Blair, M., Stewart-Brown, S., Waterston, T. and Crowther, R. (2010) *Child Public Health*, 2nd edition, Oxford: Oxford University Press.

Book Trust (2017) Dirty Bertie, retrieved from www.booktrust.org.uk/book/d/dirty-bertie (accessed 14 March 2018).

British Dental Association (2018) Oral Hygiene Resources, retrieved from www.bda.org/library/oral-hygiene (accessed 14 March 2018).

Brockman, R., Jago, R. and Fox, K. (2011) Children's Active Play: Self-reported Motivators, Barriers and Facilitators, retrieved from https://bmcpublichealth.biomedcentral. com/articles/10.1186/1471-2458-11-461 (accessed 21 March 2011).

Bruner J. (1977) *The Process of Education*, Cambridge, MA: Harvard University Press.

Bundy, D. and Horton, S. (2017) Impact of Interventions on Health and Development During Childhood and Adolescence: A Conceptual Framework, in World Bank Group, *Disease Control Priorities, Third Edition: Child and Adolescent Health and Development*, 73–78, Washington, DC: World Bank Group.

Bundy, D., de Silva, N., Horton, S., Patton, G., Schultz, L. and Jamison, D. (2017) Child and Adolescent Health and Development: Realizing Neglected Potential, in World Bank Group, *Disease Control Priorities, Third Edition: Child and Adolescent Health and Development*, 1–24, Washington, DC: World Bank Group.

Cancer Council Australia (2018) Slip Slop Slap Seek Slide, retrieved from www.cancer.org. au/preventing-cancer/sun-protection/campaigns-and-events/slip-slop-slap-seek-slide.htm l (accessed 14 March 2018).

CheesyBanana2009 (2009) Swine Flu Skank (Lyrics), retrieved from www.youtube.com/wa tch?v=SLe4m8H4qAU (accessed 16 March 2018).

Crystal, G. (2010) Preparing Your Child for Their First Dental Visit, retrieved from www.safeden tistry.co.uk/PreparingYourChildForTheirFirstDentalVisit.html (accessed 19 December 2018).

Dental Associates (2018) Traditional Braces, retrieved from www.dentalassociates.com/our-services/braces-orthodontics/traditional-braces-phase-2 (accessed 5 September 2018).

Department of Education and Childhood Development (2007) *Strategies for Improving Outcomes for Young Children: A Catalogue of Evidence-Based Interventions*, Melbourne: Victorian Government Department of Human Services.

Department of Health (2008) Swine Flu Campaign Resources, retrieved from http://weba rchive.nationalarchives.gov.uk/20130124042838/www.dh.gov.uk/prod_consum_dh/ groups/dh_digitalassets/@dh/@en/documents/digitalasset/dh_085124.pdf (accessed 19 March 2018).

Evans, K. (2018) @LancetChildAdol 'We Must Keep Engaging Young People on Solutions … Twitter, 21 February, retrieved from https://twitter.com/KathEvans2/status/ 966374551813836800 (accessed 19 March 2018).

Girl Scout Council of the Nation's Capital (2010) Sun Safety Troop Patch Program, retrieved from www.gscnc.org/content/dam/girlscouts-gscnc/documents/Kits%20and% 20Patches/Sun_Safety_patch.pdf (accessed 19 March 2018).

Fernades, M. and Aurino, E. (2017) Identifying an Essential Package for School-Aged Child Health: Economic Analysis, in World Bank Group, *Disease Control Priorities, Third Edition: Child and Adolescent Health and Development*, 355–368, Washington, DC: World Bank Group.

JuxtaPoser (2009) Swine Flu Skank (Video), 8 May, retrieved from http://djcable.blogspot. co.uk/2009/05/swine-flu-skank.html (accessed 16 March 2018).

Ladybird (2015) *Peppa Pig: Dentist Trip*. London: Penguin Books.

Kumar, S., Shaw, P., Giagkos, A., Braud, R., Lee, M. and Shen, Q. (2018) Developing Hierarchical Schemas and Building Schema Chains through Practice Play Behavior. *Frontiers in Neurorobotics*, 12: 33.

McVeigh, T. and Tuckman, J. (2009) Mexico Swine Flu Outbreak Triggers Global Pandemic Fears, *The Guardian*, retrieved from www.theguardian.com/world/2009/apr/25/ swine-flu-mexico (accessed 19 March 2018).

Marlow, B. (2015) Meet the Billion Dollar Pig Who Became the Most Important Figure in British Business, *The Telegraph*, retrieved from www.telegraph.co.uk/finance/news bysector/mediatechnologyandtelecoms/11381852/The-billion-dollar-pig-who-becam e-the-most-important-figure-in-British-business.html (accessed 17 March 2018).

Monkey Wellbeing (2018) Monkey's Guide to Healthy Teeth Pack, retrieved from www.mon keywellbeing.com/shop/monkeys-guide-to-healthy-teeth-pack (accessed 19 March 2018).

NHS Choices (2015) Braces and Orthodontics, retrieved from www.nhs.uk/Livewell/denta lhealth/Pages/braces.aspx (accessed 16 March 2018).

Ohlden, A. (2008) Dirty Bertie Dishes Tissue Advice To Mums, retrieved from www.science20. com/newswire/dirty_bertie_dishes_tissue_advice_to_mums (accessed 5 September 2018).

Online Slang Dictionary (2018) Definition of Skank, retrieved from http://onlineslangdic tionary.com/meaning-definition-of/skank (accessed 16 March 2018).

Oral Health Foundation (2016) Dental Buddy, retrieved from www.dentalbuddy.org (accessed 16 March 2018).

Perry, B., Hogan, l. and Marlin, S. (2000) Curiosity, Pleasure and Play: A Neurodevelop-mental Perspective, *HAAEYE Advocate*, August: 9–12.

Phillips, A. (2018) Learn about Braces for Kids, retrieved from www.bracesct.com/braces-for-kids (accessed 16 March 2018).

Public Health England (2015) Flu Levels Continue to Rise, retrieved from www.gov.uk/ government/news/flu-levels-continue-to-rise (accessed 14 March 2018).

RoSPA (2018) Accidents to Children, retrieved from www.rospa.com/home-safety/advice/ child-safety/accidents-to-children (accessed 14 March 2018).

Sawyer, S., Reavley, N., Bonell, C. and Patton, G. (2017) Platforms for Delivering Adolescent Health Actions, in World Bank Group, *Disease Control Priorities, Third Edition: Child and Adolescent Health and Development*, 287–305, Washington, DC: World Bank Group.

Scoop (2017) Could an Australian Seagull Have Saved a NZ Star?, retrieved from starwww. scoop.co.nz/stories/CU1712/S00096/could-an-australian-seagull-have-saved-a-nz-star. htm (accessed 16 March 2018).

Scout Association (2018a) About Us, retrieved from http://scouts.org.uk/about-us (accessed 17 March 2018).

Scout Association (2018b) What We Do, retrieved from http://scouts.org.uk/what-we-do (accessed 17 March 2018).

Scout Association (2018c) What We Do: Badges and Awards, retrieved from http://scouts. org.uk/what-we-do/badges-and-awards (accessed 17 March 2018).

Scout Association (2018d) New Research Confirms: Scouts Strengthen Communities, retrieved from http://scouts.org.uk/news/2018/01/new-research-confirms-scouts-strengthen-comm unities (accessed 17 March 2018).

Scout Association (2018e) Beavers: Health and Fitness Activity Badge, retrieved from http://members.scouts.org.uk/supportresources/4604/health-and-fitness-activity-badge/? cat=11,18,774&moduleID=10 (accessed 21 March 2018).

Scout Association (2018f) Explorers: Streets Sports Activity Badge, retrieved from http://m embers.scouts.org.uk/supportresources/4441/street-sports-activity-badge/?cat= 9,88,783&moduleID=10 (accessed 21 March 2018).

State Government of Victoria (2017) Preschoolers (3–5 Years), retrieved from www.education. vic.gov.au/childhood/parents/health/Pages/preschoolers.aspx (accessed 14 March 2018).

Sun Safe Schools (2018) About Us and Our Objectives, retrieved from www.sunsafeschools. co.uk/about (accessed 16 March 2018).

Tonkin, A. (2007) Building a Schema for Health Promotion among Pre-school Children, PhD thesis, University of Hertfordshire.

Tonkin, A. and Weldon, C. (2013) e-IRI_06_02 – X-ray: Child Development (Paediatric) e-Learning for Healthcare, retrieved from www.e-lfh.org.uk/programmes/image-interp retation (accessed 15 March 2018).

United States Environmental Protection Agency (2017) Sun Safety, retrieved from www. epa.gov/sunsafety (accessed 14 March 2018).

UproarUnltd (2009) Swine Flu Skank – The Original Track, retrieved from www.youtube.com/watch?v=npvUyxiTfYs (accessed 14 March 2018).

White, S. (2017) Health Matters: Child Dental Health, retrieved from https://publichealthmatters.blog.gov.uk/2017/06/14/health-matters-child-dental-health (accessed 3 July 2017).

Wilson, P. (1983) *Practical Dental Health Education: A Guide to Home-Made Resources and Ideas*, 2nd edition, Southern Derbyshire Health Authority.

World Bank Group (2018) *Disease Control Priorities, Third Edition: Child and Adolescent Health and Development*, Washington, DC: World Bank Group.

World Health Organization (2012) European Action Plan for Strengthening Public Health Capacities and Services, retrieved from www.euro.who.int/__data/assets/pdf_file/0005/171770/RC62wd12rev1-Eng.pdf (accessed 14 March 2018).

World Health Organization (2018a) Sun Protection, retrieved from www.who.int/uv/sun_protection/en (accessed 14 March 2018).

World Health Organization (2018b) Protecting Children, retrieved from www.who.int/uv/intersunprogramme/activities/uv_protectchildren/en (accessed 19 March 2018).

Zimmerman, E. and Woolf, S. (2014) Understanding the Relationship Between Education and Health. Discussion Paper. Institute of Medicine of the National Academies, retrieved from https://nam.edu/wp-content/uploads/2015/06/BPH-UnderstandingTheRelationship1.pdf (accessed 16 March 2018).

Zotti, F., Dalessandri, D., Salgarello, S., Piancino, M., Bonetti, S., Visconti, L. and Paganelli, C. (2016) Usefulness of an App in Improving Oral Hygiene Compliance in Adolescent Orthodontic Patients, *The Angle Orthodontist*, 86(1): 101–107.

# 9

# PLAY, DISABILITY AND PUBLIC HEALTH

*Claire Weldon and Alison Tonkin*

## Introduction

It has long been recognized that everyone should have an entitlement to basic rights and freedoms and should be treated equally with fairness, dignity and respect (Equality and Human Rights Commission 2017). However, the World Health Organization (2018a) recognizes that people with disabilities experience a greater range and number of 'unmet healthcare needs' in comparison to people who do not have a disability. The core business of public health, namely preventative action and the promotion of health, are seldom targeted at people with disabilities. Groce and Kett (2013) identify this as an example of *the disability and development gap*, whereby the lack of systematic inclusion of people with disabilities has caused them to 'lag' behind their non-disabled peers on the public health agenda. This is pertinent as people with disabilities have higher rates of engagement with risky health-related behaviors such as smoking, a lack of physical activity and poor diet (World Health Organization 2018a). These risky behaviors, together with the consumption of alcohol and being overweight, are responsible for 40 per cent of disability-adjusted life years (discussed in more detail below) in the United Kingdom (Fenton 2016). Strategic efforts to address these behaviors must incorporate the inclusion of people with disabilities in both preventative and promotional services (Centers for Disease Control and Prevention n.d.).

Public health, by its very definition, belongs to *all* the people, and aspires to '[fulfil] society's interest in assuring conditions in which people can be healthy' (Centers for Disease Control and Prevention n.d.). The centrality of society's communal efforts to secure optimal conditions to enable everyone to live a healthy life echoes the original definition of public health by Winslow (1920: 30) whereby 'organized community efforts' were regarded as the means to 'enable every citizen to realize his birth-right of health and longevity'. The scope of public health practice needs to reflect the inclusivity inherent in this statement, by addressing the social inequalities linked to health as part of its mission (Berghs et al. 2017).

Article 25 of the United Nations Convention on the Rights of Persons with Disabilities (CRPD) (United Nations 2017) states that people with disabilities 'have the right to the enjoyment of the highest attainable standard of health without discrimination on the basis of disability' and this includes 'population-based public health programmes'. The Equality and Human Rights Commission (2017) suggest that Article 25 should not be understood as 'a right to health' but as a right to the facilitation to achieve the best possible health. Acknowledging the interconnectedness and reciprocity of the rights within the CRPD, Article 30 identifies the right of people with disabilities to 'access and participate in cultural life, recreation, leisure and sport (ibid.), with all the health-related benefits associated with these activities (APPG on Arts, Health and Wellbeing 2017; Public Health England 2016). This chapter will focus on the exploration of play and playfulness as a means of enhancing the fulfilment of Articles 25 and 30, by making optimal use of available resources to improve health outcomes for all (World Health Organization 2018a).

## Defining 'disability'

One billion people, or 15 per cent of the global population, have 'some sort of disability' and the incidence is increasing, in part due to an aging population but also due to an increase in chronic health conditions (World Health Organization 2018a). With such a high level of prevalence, a broad definition of 'some sort of disability' is necessary if it is to reflect the impact of disability on the individuals concerned.

The World Health Organization (2018b) define disability as 'an umbrella term', which covers:

- Impairments – 'a problem in bodily function or structure'.
- Activity limitations – 'difficulty encountered by an individual in executing a task or action'.
- Participation restrictions – 'a problem experienced by an individual in involvement in life situations'.

The Equality Act 2010, which applies across the UK, describes a person with a disability as 'someone who has a physical or mental impairment which has a substantial and long-term [lasting at least 12 months] adverse effect on their ability to carry out normal day-to-day activities' (Department for Work and Pensions and Department of Health and Social Care 2017).

Learning disabilities, which affect a person for the whole of their lives, reduce intellectual capacity and make certain everyday activities more difficult, such as managing money, household tasks or socializing (Mencap 2018). In comparison to the general population, people with learning disabilities have poorer health, much of which could be prevented (Public Health England 2018). Difficulties in getting effective and timely healthcare have serious consequences, leading to a poorer quality of life (ibid.).

It is important that definitions of disability incorporate the lived experience of people affected, so that society can respond in an appropriate manner to meet their needs. The impact of disability on health can be measured through the concept of the 'disability-adjusted life year' (DALY), which describes the global burden of disease on people living with a disability (Public Health England 2015). DALYs 'add the years of life lost due to early death, and years spent living with disability or ill-health, together' (ibid.). They are calculated for a wide range of diseases and injuries and are based on presumptions about the service adjustments necessary in response to the physical or mental disability, allowing for age-related variables (Fox-Rushby 2002).

Disability, whatever form it takes, prevents people from having equal choices and chances to participate and engage with all that society has to offer. These societal barriers can be categorized as:

- physical or environmental – ones that we can touch or see;
- social or attitudinal – the way people think and act;
- organizational, financial and even emotional. *(Disability Arts Cymru 2018)*

## Society's perception of disability

Societal attitudes have been identified as a major causative factor of disability for people with impairments. Public perceptions of disability are attributed as 'the roots of discrimination and the causes of social exclusion' (Disability Arts Cymru 2018). Cultural traditions and historical beliefs still influence practices and perceptions in the modern era and Blunkett (2015) acknowledges that, while some progress has been made in recent years, public perceptions of disability need to change further if we are to address the social exclusion of people with disabilities.

In the 1970s and 1980s, *disabled activists* developed the Social Model of Disability as a means of reflecting their personal experiences of disability (Disability Arts Cymru 2018). The Social Model of Disability states that it is the *organization of society*, rather than individual impairments or differences, that limits a person's sensory, physical or mental function and ultimately 'creates' the disability (Scope 2017). This suggests that it is society which has created the barriers which restrict life-choices for people with disabilities, and that it is by removing these barriers that 'disabled people can be independent and equal in society, with choice and control over their own lives' (ibid.).

Blunkett (2015) advocates an approach which promotes people's ability to engage with, and participate in, their community with all the associated benefits to wellbeing. Figure 9.1 illustrates the barriers associated with the physical environment of a theatre, for example. Instead of focusing on the 'individual' as the problem, a social model of disability focuses on the assessment and adaptation of environmental barriers to cultural inclusion (A Guide to Theatre Access 2017).

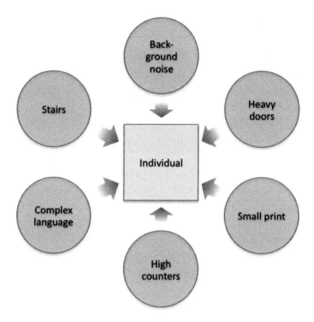

**FIGURE 9.1** The Social Model of Disability linked to environmental barriers.
Source: A Guide to Theatre Access (2017)

This approach is summarized by Disability Arts Cymru (2018), who state that 'What matters is an understanding that people may have different ways of accessing things, but by working together, we can make huge changes for the better. Every single thing you do to improve access will make a difference.'

Since the introduction of the social model of disability, there have been many changes across the world in terms of the relative status of people with disabilities and how they are treated within society. The social model of disability is regarded as a powerful tool in relation to policy, planning and subsequent practice. By identifying and removing barriers, this approach promotes access and engagement for people with disabilities (A Guide to Theatre Access 2017). For example, Microsoft has become the first major gaming company to develop a marketable product that enables gamers with disabilities to access video games (Stuart 2018). The Xbox adaptive controller 'features two large buttons for hands, elbows or feet, as well as 19 ports to accommodate extra devices including mouth-operated "sip and puff" quadsticks' (Stuart 2018). Developed collaboratively with occupational therapists, gamers with a range of disabilities, and charities such the Cerebral Palsy Foundation and the veterans' organization Warfighter Engaged, the adaptive controller represents an accessible and affordable gadget (Stuart 2018) which 'will send out a message to lots of people who have a disability, that "I can actually join in with everyone else" and … this [inclusivity] is one of the most important aspects of this product' (Donegan cited in Powell 2018).

## Advocacy and action

In 2006, following 20 years of campaigning by people with disabilities, the United Nations Convention on the Rights of Persons with Disabilities (UNCRPD) was introduced (United Nations 2018). This is an international agreement which aims to 'set out the steps which every country in the world should take to remove these obstacles [to participate in society] and… to drive forward real dignity, equality and inclusion for disabled people' (Equality and Human Rights Commission 2017: 6). Ultimately, it is the role of society which is key to changing attitudes to disability. This is noted by the Equality and Human Rights Commission (ibid.: 27), who state: 'Disabled people can enjoy full human rights only if society changes its attitude towards disabled people. This won't happen by itself.'

The remainder of this chapter will explore a range of play-based projects and approaches that exemplify the identification and minimization of societal barriers to inclusion, resulting in opportunities for people with impairments to engage with all the health and wellbeing benefits associated with playful pursuits (Equality and Human Rights Commission 2017).

## Equality and non-discrimination – Article 5 (UNCRPD)

Article 5 highlights the premise that everyone is equal under the law and that discrimination against people with disabilities is not allowed (EasyRead 2007). As noted earlier, the rights within the UNCRPD are interrelated and mutually inclusive. The Equality and Human Rights Commission (2017) provides the following worked example of how Article 5 can be applied in relation to Article 30: the right to participate in leisure activities:

> A local authority decides to close a car park which gives easy access to a beach, resulting in visitors having to park further away and to use an alternative route which is steep. This means that people with mobility impairments and their family/friends cannot go to that beach anymore. This is a regressive step and also it puts disabled people at a disadvantage in comparison with other people. Disabled people could highlight Articles 5 and 30 in their discussions with, or a case against, the local authority in such a situation.
>
> *(Equality and Human Rights Commission 2017: 24)*

This example also exposes the value of raising *awareness* (Article 8), which provides an opportunity for people to reflect on the impact of decision-making, which may not have been previously considered. It also raises the issue of *accessibility* (Article 9), in this instance, access to the physical environment. All people should have an *opportunity* to be involved in the life of their community (Article 19). This example highlights how people with a disability may be denied the opportunity to engage with an aspect of the community, limiting independent *mobility* (Article 20).

Restricted mobility may also be overcome through innovative action, such as the introduction of beach wheelchairs. In 2015, a Scottish company Beach Wheelchairs (2017) introduced specially designed, highly mobile, wheelchairs which have large rubber wheels that can be move easily over sand. Available for hire at a number of beach locations in North Berwick, beach wheelchairs can enable wheelchair-users to enjoy a family day out at the seaside with the associated benefits to physical, social and emotional health: 'For the first time since her accident Sarah could go down to the beach with her husband, kids and dog and have an amazing time. She even dipped her toe in the sea!' (Beach Wheelchairs 2017).

## Awareness raising – Article 8 (UNCRPD)

Article 8 is fundamental for changing perceptions of disability, and governments are urged to 'raise awareness throughout society, including at family level, and to encourage respect towards disabled people' (Equality and Human Rights Commission 2017: 27).

Public health campaigns are aimed at preventing illness and disease in the general population, but few government campaigns acknowledge the specific needs of individuals with disabilities or long-term health conditions. In contrast, the third sector, which includes special interest groups who advocate for specific health related conditions and their associated impairments, has mounted various targeted campaigns. The best way to 'raise awareness' is to foster inclusive attitudes from an early age and the Yard (2016) in Eastern Scotland offers disabled children, young people and their siblings opportunities to engage in 'creative, adventurous indoor and outdoor play in a well-supported environment'. Families who utilize the services describe them as a 'lifeline that creates a sense of belonging, community and support for parents and carers too' (Yard 2016).

Time to Change, led by the mental health charities Mind and Rethink, aims to end mental health discrimination, producing a variety of resources for schools which include games, witty adverts and posters (see www.time-to-change.org.uk). These resources use play as a means of engagement to increase awareness around mental health issues, to reduce stigma, and to direct individuals towards appropriate support.

The Scout Association (2018), which caters for boys and girls aged six to 25 years of age, highlights the fact that, unless young people have a family member or friend with a disability, they may not have the opportunity to learn about disability. Scouting provides age-appropriate resources, including dedicated Disability Awareness badges for the younger age sections (Beavers and Cubs) and activities for all sections which help young people 'to be more empathetic and understanding adults in the future'. All sections are encouraged to work towards:

- exploring and clarifying what 'being disabled' means;
- learning how it can affect people; and
- taking action to make the local community more friendly and accessible.

Dedicated scouting campaigns such as A Million Hands, incorporate suggested activities which can be factored into the planning of weekly meetings across the section (Scout Association 2016). The playing of games is a recognized experiential learning opportunity. For example, 'Getting from A to B' involves young people navigating a simple obstacle course in pairs, with one of the pair blindfolded and the other acting as 'guide'. They are later invited to discuss the difficulties they encountered, and this discussion can be expanded to a broader consideration of relevant issues in relation to other types of disability (Scout Association 2016).

Stickman Communications provides a 'refreshing, stylish, light-hearted yet true-to-life approach to disability' (Stickman Communications 2018a). 'Resources have been developed from personal experience of disability using humor to portray life with a disability as a "differently normal" thing' (Stickman Communications 2018b). The creator has developed a range of resources 'using stickmen and simple phrases' to 'help break down barriers, challenge preconceptions, promote understanding and acceptance, and enable communication' (see http://stickmancommunications.co.uk). The resources include communication cards (Figure 9.2) that explain conditions and situations from the perspective of the card carrier. These allow people with disabilities or impairments to communicate non-verbally, by presenting the card rather than struggling to verbalize their needs.

Podcasts (downloadable digital audio files on the internet) are a way of raising awareness of disability issues for all sectors of the population. The British Broadcasting Corporation (BBC) produces regular podcasts about disability, health and mental health. The *Ouch: Disability Talk* (BBC 2018) podcast, features guests discussing a range of disability-related topics in a personal and humorous manner. The discussions are an opportunity to raise awareness about the issues affecting individuals with disabilities and long-term health conditions and those who support them. Often using irreverent humor to discuss intimate topics, examples include the Valentine-themed podcast on 2 February 2018 entitled 'Love me, love my wheels?' which 'expose[d] the less known side of canoodling for disabled people' (BBC 2018). The podcasts also address health-related topics, such as the instalment on 12 January 2018 which asked: 'Is it harder for disabled people to lose weight?' This instalment also featured the 'lowdown on wheelchair spinning classes and awkward hospital moments' (ibid.).

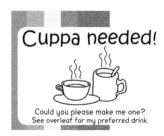

**FIGURE 9.2** Example communication card.
Source: reproduced by kind permission of Stickman Communications

The importance of exercise and physical activity for physical and mental health is well documented (Disability Rights UK 2017) but the opportunities for active play and exercise are more limited for people with disabilities. Pollard (n.d.), citing a survey by Sport England, identified that four out of five people with a disability report taking little or no exercise, although this was not through personal choice. Research undertaken by the English Federation of Disability Sport (Spring 2014) identifies the importance of communication in increasing the awareness of disability sport, suggesting that it is important to utilize a variety of communication formats so that the widest range of individuals can be reached regardless of their disability status.

Spring (2014) further suggests that most barriers to inclusion are related to personal confidence and the responses of other people. This is particularly important for children with a disability as 'the early attainment of motor and social skills' is essential for subsequent engagement with physical activity (Shields and Synnot 2016). Children with disabilities are less likely to engage in physical activity in comparison to children on typical developmental pathways, and reasons cited include 'a lack of instructor skills and unwillingness to be inclusive, negative societal attitudes towards disability, and a lack of local opportunities' (ibid.). Although the barriers to engagement have been studied more than the facilitators, Shields and Synnot identify the following factors:

- the child's desire to be fit and active
- skills practice
- involvement of peers
- family support
- close and accessible facilities
- opportunities sensitive to the needs to children with disability
- skilled staff
- information dissemination.*(Shields and Synnot 2016)*

The Yard (2016) addresses all these facilitators and provides a model example of how to provide an inclusive play environment that promotes risk and challenge for all children and young people, including those with disabilities and impairments. Inclusive play enhances self-esteem, confidence and emotional wellbeing.

## Accessibility – Article 9 (UNCRPD)

This article requires countries to 'make sure disabled people have better access to things in all areas of life' (EasyRead 2007: 10).

As noted previously, the Social Model of Disability can be used to promote accessibility, enabling everybody 'to freely participate in the cultural life of the community … yet when people become disabled or marginalised because of ill health, life opportunities can decrease significantly' (Dementia and Imagination 2017).

In 2005, the charity Barnardos undertook an evaluation of a £10.8 million, four-year project called the Better Play Programme (Ludvigsen et al. 2005). Re-asserting that inclusive play means that *all* children should be included in play opportunities, irrespective of whether they have a disability, the evaluation identified many barriers that needed to be overcome before a definition of 'inclusive play' could be justified (ibid.). The barriers identified included environmental factors, such as a lack of physical access, as well as attitudinal and social barriers. The report noted that, while it was not realistic to expect that all children will always be able to participate in all activities, inclusive play should ensure that all children have a 'real choice of play activities' (ibid.).

Ten years after the Barnardos study, Sense (2015) the national disability charity for people with complex communication needs, undertook a Public Inquiry that focused on the provision of play opportunities for children with multiple needs in the 0-five years age group. It clearly showed that, while the provision of play opportunities for children with complex needs is vital, there were significant barriers to accessing high quality play provision (ibid.). As a result, Sense (2018a) have produced a variety of play toolkits that are differentiated for parents or professionals and which 'provide information and advice on enabling children with complex communication needs to enjoy inclusive play' (ibid.). The toolkits have been produced in collaboration with the parents of children who have complex needs and 'contain simple ideas, suggestions and practical tips on making play fun and fully accessible' (ibid.).

Sense (2018b) also advocates for people to be able to participate in physical activity and to express themselves creatively throughout the life-course, irrespective of the complexity of their needs. Sense perceives their role as: 'a driver for social change, influencing the arts and social care sectors through high quality inclusive arts practice':

> *Sense Art* promotes 'pioneering sensory arts activities'
> *Sense Sports* works in partnership with Sports England to run sport and physical activity events
> *Sense Wellbeing* combines the best of both the arts and sports programs to promote wellbeing and improve quality of life.
>
> *(Sense 2018b)*

The Dementia & Imagination Project (2017) explored how art could improve life for people with dementia and their carers. The aim was to assess whether art helped the individual to stay connected with their community and whether the community could become more dementia friendly. The project involved weekly creative art sessions led by artists for groups of individuals who may or may not have dementia. The participants did not need any prior experience or knowledge of the arts and the intention was to offer 'meaningful engagement, stimulating imagination and discussion… to encourage creativity…be interesting and challenging, and promote learning where possible' (Dementia and Imagination 2017). The artists were encouraged to adapt the sessions to meet the needs of individual participants with the aim of developing wellbeing, self-expression and pleasure and encouraging interpersonal connection.

A further example of innovative practice for improving accessibility is the concept of *Touch Tours*. Touch tours have been developed to enable those with sensory impairments to access museums and the artefacts on display. The American Museum of Natural History (2018) offers Science Scene Tours for people with visual impairments, where 'specially trained Museum tour guides highlight specific themes and exhibits, engaging participants through extensive verbal descriptions and touchable objects'. The San Antonio Museum of Art 'offers guided tours of the galleries, and includes touch, verbal descriptions, sounds, and even smells!' (Stalvey 2015). The British Museum (2018) provides tailored sessions for children with additional needs, enabling them to 'experience ancient Greece, Egypt, the Vikings, Roman Britain or medieval Britain through sight, sound, smell and touch with these facilitated sessions', while the Australian Museum provides materials with large print or Braille, tactile drawings, audio description and guided tours as part of the drive to 'focus on social and physical inclusion rather than disability' (Australian Museum 2018).

## Habilitation and rehabilitation – Article 26 (UNCRPD)

Article 26 relates to the development of skills to facilitate independent living and support to participate in the community. Habilitation is the learning of new skills that have not been learnt before, while rehabilitation refers to the re-learning of a skill, such as talking or walking (Equality and Human Rights Commission 2017).

InstructAbility is a scheme that 'provides disabled people with free, accessible fitness industry training and qualifications followed by a voluntary industry work placement. By supporting disabled people to take up a fitness career, we can help to encourage other disabled people in the local community to access leisure facilities, participate in inclusive fitness activities and enjoy an active lifestyle' (Aspire 2018). This scheme has multiple benefits. Firstly, people with disabilities can acquire new skills and gain qualifications which nurture the development of confidence and self-esteem, as well as offering a route to financial independence. Secondly, once participants have gained the necessary qualifications they are in a position to encourage others with disabilities to participate in sport. Sport 'increases social opportunities and community involvement, as well as opening up voluntary and training opportunities such as coaching' (Inspire Peterborough 2018). There follow three examples of individuals who have used their own experience of physical and sporting achievement as motivation for helping others with disabilities to enjoy 'getting physical'.

Jonnie Peacock, the English sprint runner and Paralympics gold medal winner, participated in a campaign by the Papworth Trust and Living Sport and Ability Plus, to encourage people with disabilities to take part in sport. Peacock states that sport helped him during his teenage years and that he now wants to encourage other people to experience the benefits that sport can offer.

Tennis coach Oli Jones was diagnosed with bipolar disorder in adulthood and found that exercise helped him to manage his symptoms:

> Being active kick-starts the body into releasing endorphins, our natural, mood-lifting chemicals. Endorphins restrict the body's pain signal transmission, and they create a feeling of euphoria…So every time you go for a run, swim, row, walk, gym session…you are quite literally giving your body and brain a better chance to feel much better.
>
> *(Jones 2015)*

The founder of Wheely Good Fitness (2018), Kris Saunders-Stowe is a wheelchair user and has developed exercise classes and DVD resources to encourage individuals to take part in physical activities they enjoy. When exercising or training in a wheelchair, the use of the body is very different and fitness activities need to reflect this difference (ibid.). With a focus on the development of fitness activities tailored to individual need, the Wheely Good Fitness programme allows wheelchair users to develop new skills while doing something that reinforces learning through the pleasure pathways.

These examples demonstrate the many opportunities to increase participation in community activities and encapsulated in the following statement by *Doing Sport Differently* (Disability Rights 2017): 'Millions of players, thousands of activities, endless possibilities'.

## Participation in cultural life, recreation, leisure and sport –

### Article 30 (UNCRPD)

Governments are required to support people with disabilities to participate on an equal basis and advocacy for play and playful activities is essential for inclusive participation in all aspects of social and cultural life.

In 2017, the All Party Parliamentary Group on Arts, Health and Wellbeing's inquiry report was published. This substantial publication, covering 192 pages, provides a comprehensive overview of how the arts contribute to health and wellbeing. The report is evidence-based and provides a wealth of examples of the health benefits of music, singing, dance, visual and digital arts, film, performing arts, the written and spoken word and community festivals (APPG on Arts, Health and Wellbeing 2017). Disability and the Arts are reflected throughout the report which advocates for all people to have opportunities to engage with the creative arts as a means of promoting health and wellbeing. With so many examples of flexible and innovative approaches to engaging people with disabilities, this report provides a rich source of inspiration that acknowledges the 'creative impulse is fundamental to the experience of being human' (ibid.: 10).

## Conclusion

There are many opportunities for individuals with disabilities or long-term health conditions to engage in play and sporting activities. However, there is still a need to challenge perceptions of disability and to increase opportunities for inclusive participation in play and recreation. Blunkett (2015) suggests that 'disabled or not, all of us are dependent on the mutuality and reciprocity which are the hallmarks of a civilized society at some time of our lives. And isn't a civilized society the kind of society we all want to live in?'.

## References

A Guide to Theatre Access (2017) A Note on the Social Model of Disability, retrieved from www.accessibletheatre.org.uk/senior-managers/a-note-on-the-social-model-of-disability (accessed 4 December 2017).

American Museum of Natural History (2018) Science Sense Tours, retrieved from www.am nh.org/plan-your-visit/accessibility (accessed 7 May 2018).

APPG on Arts, Health and Wellbeing (2017) *Creative Health: The Arts for Health and Wellbeing* [The Short Report], London: All Party Parliamentary Group on Arts, Health and Wellbeing.

Aspire (2018) InstructAbility, retrieved from www.aspire.org.uk/instructability (accessed 5 September 2018).

Australian Museum (2018) *Accessibility and Inclusion Action Plan 2018–2021: Providing Accessible and Inclusive Exhibits, Programs and Services*, Sydney: Australian Museum.

BBC (2018) Ouch: Disability Talk: Podcast, retrieved from www.bbc.co.uk/programmes/p 02r6yqw/episodes/downloads (accessed 5 April 2018).

Beach Wheelchairs (2017) About Us, retrieved from www.beachwheelchairs.org (accessed 13 May 2018).

Berghs, M., Atkin, K., Graham, H., Hatton, C. and Thomas, C. (2017) Public Health, Research and Rights: The Perspectives of Deliberation Panels with Politically and Socially Active Disabled People, *Disability & Society*, 32(7), 945–965.

Blunkett, D. (2015) The Public's Perception of Disabled People Needs to Change – We're Not Just Paralympians or Scroungers, *The Independent*, 12 March, retrieved from www.indep endent.co.uk/voices/comment/the-publics-perception-of-disabled-people-needs-to-change-were-not-just-paralympians-or-scroungers-10104704.html (accessed 5 September 2018).

British Museum (2018) Access and SEN Inclusive Learning Opportunities for All Young Visitors, retrieved from www.britishmuseum.org/learning/schools_and_teachers/access_a nd_sen.aspx (accessed 7 May 2018).

Centers for Disease Control and Prevention (n.d.) Public Health 101 Series: Introduction to Public Health, retrieved from www.cdc.gov/publichealth101/documents/introduction-to-public-health.pdf (accessed 13 November 2017).

Dementia and Imagination (2017) *Research Informed Approaches to Visual Arts Programmes*, Dementia and Imagination.

Department for Work and Pensions and Department of Health and Social Care (2017) Consultation Outcome: Work, Health and Disability Green Paper: Improving Lives, retrieved from www.gov.uk/government/consultations/work-health-and-disability-improving-lives/work-health-and-disability-green-paper-improving-lives (accessed 24 March 2018).

Disability Arts Cymru (2018) Society and Disabled People: Background and History, retrieved from www.disabilityartscymru.co.uk/equal-spaces/equal-spaces-background-to-disability-issues/society-and-disabled-people (accessed 24 March 2018).

Disability Rights UK (2017) *Doing Sport Differently: A Guide to Exercise and Fitness for People Living with Disability or Health Conditions*, Disability Rights UK.

EasyRead (2007) *International Agreement on the Rights of Disabled People: EasyRead Version*, Inspired Services Publishing.

Equality and Human Rights Commission (2017) *The United Nations Convention on the Rights of Persons with Disabilities: What Does It Mean for You?*, Equality and Human Rights Commission.

Fenton, K. (2016) Our Support for Population behaviour Change, retrieved from https://publichealthmatters.blog.gov.uk/2016/09/02/our-support-for-population-behaviour-change (accessed 13 November 2017).

Fox-Rushby, J. (2002) *Disability Adjusted Life Years (DALYs) for Decision Making? An Overview of the Literature*, London: Office of Health Economics.

Groce, N. and Kett, M. (2013) *The Disability and Development Gap*, London: Leonard Cheshire Disability and Inclusive Development Centre, University College London.

Inspire Peterborough (2018) Jonnie Peacock Encourages Disabled People to Enjoy Sport, retrieved from www.inspirepeterborough.com/jonnie-peacock-encourages-disabled-people-to-enjoy-sport/ (accessed 9 January 2018).

Jones, O. (2015) Centre Court for Mental Health, retrieved from www.mind.org.uk/information-support/your-stories/centre-court-for-mental-health/#.WkUDHk1LHIV (accessed 5 September 2018).

Ludvigsen, A., Creegan, C. and Mills, H. (2005) Let's Play Together: Play and Inclusion. Evaluation of Better Play Round Three, retrieved from www.barnardos.org.uk/lets_play_together_report.pdf (accessed 5 April 2018).

Mencap (2018) What Is Learning Disability?, retrieved from www.mencap.org.uk/learning-disability-explained/what-learning-disability (accessed 25 March 2018).

Pollard, J. (n.d.) Being Active: An Everyday Guide for People Living with an Impairment or Health Condition, retrieved from www.efds.co.uk/assets/000/000/149/2518_BeingActiveReport_A4_FINAL%281%29_original.pdf?1461165840 (accessed 5 January 2018).

Powell, S. (2018) Xbox Controller a 'First' for Disabled Gamers, retrieved from www.bbc.co.uk/news/av/newsbeat-44150653/xbox-adaptive-controller-a-first-for-disabled-gamers (accessed 18 May 2018).

Public Health England (2015) GBD Compare: A New Data Tool for Professionals, retrieved from https://publichealthmatters.blog.gov.uk/2015/09/15/gbd-compare-a-new-data-tool-for-professionals (accessed 5 April 2018).

Public Health England (2016) Guidance: Health Matters: Getting Every Adult Active Every Day, retrieved from www.gov.uk/government/publications/health-matters-getting-every-adult-active-every-day/health-matters-getting-every-adult-active-every-day (accessed 13 November 2017).

Public Health England (2018) Learning Disability Profiles: Introduction, retrieved from https://fingertips.phe.org.uk/profile/learning-disabilities (accessed 25 March 2018).

Sense (2015) *Making the Case for Play*, Sense.

Sense (2018a) Making Play Inclusive, retrieved from www.sense.org.uk/get-support/information-and-advice/support-for-children/play-toolkits (accessed 5 April 2018).

Sense (2018b) Arts, Sport and Wellbeing, retrieved from www.sense.org.uk/get-support/arts-sport-and-wellbeing (accessed 5 April 2018).

Scope (2017) The Social Model of Disability, retrieved from www.scope.org.uk/about-us/our-brand/social-model-of-disability (accessed 3 December 2017).

Scout Association (2016) A Million Hands | Disability Activities to Do With Your Section, 11 March, retrieved from http://scouts.org.uk/news/2016/03/a-million-hands-disability-activities-to-do-with-your-section (accessed 5 April 2018).

Scout Association (2018) What We Do, retrieved from https://scouts.org.uk/what-we-do (accessed 5 September 2018).

Stalvey, M. (2015) 8 Awesome Museums with 'Touch Tours' for Visitors who are Blind or Visually Impaired, 29 June, retrieved from https://curlabilityblog.com/2015/06/29/8-a wesome-museums-touch-tours-blind-visually-impaired (accessed 7 May 2018).

Stickman Communications (2018a) Stickman Communications, retrieved from http:// stickmancommunications.co.uk/epages/747384.sf/en_GB/?ObjectPath=/Shops/747384/ Categories (accessed 16 April 2018).

Stickman Communications (2018b) About Us, retrieved from http://stickmancommunica tions.co.uk/epages/747384.sf/en_GB/?ObjectPath=/Shops/747384/Categories/About_ Us (accessed 5 April 2018).

Shields, N. and Synnot, A. (2016) Perceived Barriers and Facilitators to Participation in Physical Activity for Children with Disability: A Qualitative Study, *BMC Pediatrics*, 16 (2016): 9.

Spring, E. (2014) *Active Together: Evidence-Based Report on How to Provide Sport or Physical Activity Opportunities for Disabled and Non-disabled People to Take Part Together*, English Federation of Disability Sport.

Stuart, K. (2018) Microsoft to Launch Disability-Friendly Xbox Controller, *The Guardian*, 17 May, retrieved from www.theguardian.com/games/2018/may/17/microsoft-xbox-disabili ty-friendly-adaptive-controller (accessed 18 May 2018).

United Nations (2017) Article 25 – Health, retrieved from www.un.org/development/desa/ disabilities/convention-on-the-rights-of-persons-with-disabilities/article-25-health.html (accessed 13 November 2017).

United Nations (2018) Convention on the Rights of Persons with Disabilities (CRPD), retrieved from www.un.org/development/desa/disabilities/convention-on-the-rights-of-p ersons-with-disabilities.html (accessed 2 May 2018).

Wheely Good Fitness (2018) About, retrieved from https://wheelygoodfitness.com (accessed 7 May 2018).

Winslow, C. (1920) The Untilled Fields of Public Health, *Science* 51(1306): 23–33.

World Health Organization (2018a) Media Centre: Disability and Health, retrieved from www.who.int/mediacentre/factsheets/fs352/en (accessed 24 March 2018).

World Health Organization (2018b) Health Topics: Disabilities, retrieved from www.who. int/topics/disabilities/en (accessed 24 October 2017).

Yard (2016) What We Believe In, retrieved from www.theyardscotland.org.uk/who-we-a re-and-what-we-believe-in (accessed 13 May 2018).

# 10

# A PLAYFUL WORKING LIFE AND BEYOND

*Christina Freeman and Alison Tonkin*

## Introduction

Public Health England (2018) states that 'employment is a primary determinant of health, impacting both directly and indirectly on the individual, their families and communities'. This designates the workplace as a prime arena for public health activity, and full employment as a key political goal designed to enable everyone to 'enjoy the independence, security and good health that being in work can bring' (Department for Work and Pensions and Department of Health 2016).

Marmot (2010: 20) states that 'being in good employment is protective of health' and this provides benefits for both mental and physical health (Black 2016). Conversely, unemployment contributes to poor health (Institute of Health Equality 2018) with financial implications not only for the individual concerned, but also for the wider economy. Absence from work, and unemployment due to long-term sickness, cost UK business approximately £15 billion a year (Black 2016).

In England, 74 per cent of the adult population are presently in employment, spending on average a third of their waking hours working (Public Health England 2018). The nature of our work defines us as individuals, contributing not only to how well we live but also to how long we live (TUC 2010). There is a growing body of evidence to demonstrate that active, engaged, and healthy employees are more productive and have lower levels of absenteeism and presenteeism (Public Health England 2018). Although employment *per se* is important for promoting health and wellbeing, the quality of employment is also a major contributory factor 'in helping people to stay healthy and happy, something which benefits people and serves the wider public interest' (Taylor 2017: 6).

The role of play and playfulness in the workplace is increasingly seen as a means of encouraging creativity and innovation, as well as of enhancing motivation, commitment and job satisfaction (Everett 2011). As Bradshaw (2013) suggests:

> We often think of play and work as separate. But we need to be more willing to let our minds play while working. Think about it. How often do you leave work with the solution to a problem just out of reach? You might walk the dog, go to the gym or meet a friend for coffee and – while your mind is 'at play' – the answer arrives in a flash of inspiration, a moment of clarity.

A playful mindset benefits both the employer and the employee and, for the organization, workplace fun is an inexpensive and profitable means of engagement which cultivates morale (Everett 2011). Everett (2011: 1) makes the important distinction between 'manufactured' and 'organic' fun, the latter being identified as 'a descendent of a positive organizational culture [that] will thrive in the most diverse workplaces'. This chapter will explore the role of 'organic fun' within the context of *good work* and organizational culture, both of which contribute to the development of relationships between the worker and the organization and to the promotion of good physical and mental health (TUC 2010). It will conclude by reviewing how playful strategies can be used to facilitate the transition into retirement and beyond, creating continuity between the behaviors and dispositions of a working life and new experiences in later life (Payson 2019).

## Conceptualizing good work and play

One of Marmot's six policy objectives from the classic report *Fair Society, Healthy Lives* was the need to 'create fair employment and good work for all' (Local Government Association 2018). The phrase *good work* has a specific meaning that dates from 1971 when the Swedish Trade Union Federation instigated a debate with the government and with employers about the link between the work environment and democracy (TUC 2010: 4). Although there are a variety of definitions associated with the concept of *good work*, the basic premise is that work should be organized in a way that actively promotes good physical and mental health (ibid.).

In 2017, the Taylor Review identified seven steps 'towards fair and decent work', one of which stated that 'the shape and content of work and individual health and well-being are strongly related. For the benefit for firms, workers and the public interest we need to develop a more proactive approach to workplace health' (Taylor 2017: 111). Play and playfulness are recognized for their ability to promote good physical and mental health (van Vleet and Feeney 2015) and it is therefore apposite to discuss the concepts of *good work* and play as they relate to each other.

The term *a playful workforce* evokes images of the trendy new work environments of social media and advertising organizations, which promote the use play as part of their business model (Pflug and Jara 2014). Among the most popular examples of play in the workplace are computer gaming and indoor physical recreation such as table tennis. The theory underpinning such a break from the traditional work environment suggests that playing in the workplace simply makes for happier, more creative and more productive staff (Everett 2011) but workplace gamification is also becoming an essential tool in the 'corporate toolbox' (Pflug and Jara 2014).

Workplace gamification systems which use game thinking and game dynamics to develop skills, promote learning, and change behavior, have been predicted to grow rapidly in the next few years. Research shows that more than 1,400 global organizations already employ gamification applications (Pflug and Jara 2014).

While acknowledging the success of such playful endeavors in the corporate sphere, it may seem incongruous to advocate play and playfulness in the more traditional context of the public sector: in education, health and social care. Yet, the notorious use of dark humor often associated with those working in the emergency services is known to be a protective practice which can provide emotional release when dealing with difficult, deeply unpleasant, and sometimes life-threatening situations (Charman, cited in University of Portsmouth 2013). Research from the University of Portsmouth (2013) suggests that 'black humor drawn from shared experiences, helps "glue" ambulance crews and police officers together, with firefighters likely to be on the receiving end of the jokes'. Dark gallows humor is often described by those who use it as 'inappropriate, warped, bizarre and slightly sick', and Charman (cited in University of Portsmouth 2013) goes on to explain that 'risqué humor demands a high degree of trust and confidence between colleagues and has the potential to be career threatening, but the humor between ambulance crews and police officers is seen by them as unremittingly positive'. As with many other areas of employment, such as academia and education, retail, catering, business, social care and the justice system, what makes colleagues laugh is culturally defined, based on shared experiences at work and the nature of the work itself (University of Portsmouth 2013).

## Play within the organizational context

Within the modern context of acknowledging wellbeing and mental wellness as features of good work, there is an increasing desire to foster a culture within the workplace which is altogether kinder and more sensitive to the needs and personal potential of the individual (NHS Leadership Academy 2013). Immersion in games and playful pursuits enables people to feel relaxed, often revealing skills or dispositions that may otherwise lay dormant (gamelearn 2018).

According to van Vleet and Feeney (cited in Minds for Business 2017), play can be defined as: 'a behavior or activity carried out with the goal of amusement and fun', which 'involves an enthusiastic and in-the-moment attitude or approach', and 'is highly interactive among play partners or with the activity itself'.

Play in the context of the workplace demands special consideration of the power differences that are inherent in the setting, due to the nature of the work being performed and the workforce itself, as well as the unique culture of the organization (Minds for Business 2017). Most people work within a structured employment model and the way the organization functions may be described as a work culture. The culture of any organization is inherently complex. It can be viewed from multiple perspectives and can reflect various overlapping dimensions (Businessballs 2017). The nature of the work culture can foster 'discovery and invention'

(Csikszentmihalyi 2009) or it can stifle creativity and innovation (Taylor 2016) and this difference will impact on how play and playfulness are perceived, or even tolerated, within the organization.

In 1978, Charles Handy published *Gods of Management: The Changing Work of Organizations*, which explored how organizations function as a consequence of human behaviors and organizational structure. Handy used stories from ancient Greek mythology and drawings to playfully explore organizational cultures, suggesting that 'management is more fun, more creative, more personal, more political and more intuitive than any textbook' (Handy 1978: 4). Using patterns of human behavior that could be categorized into practical models, Handy classified four differing cultures (as described in Table 10.1), each one describing an individual's function and role within the organization (ProvenModels 2018). Handy believed that each of these cultures co-exists within an organization, meaning that any intervention or change needs to strike a balance between them if they are to be effective.

## Role cultures

Handy identified organizations as role-based cultures when they were founded on rules. Everyone in the organization knows what their roles and responsibilities are, and the power of an individual is determined by their place in the organizational structure. Organizations with role cultures tend to have a long chain of command, which often makes decision-making slow. It seems that playfulness within this sort

**TABLE 10.1** Organizational cultures described by Handy.

| Culture | God | Key features |
|---|---|---|
| Role | Apollo | Power is hierarchical – efficiency comes from adherence to order. Decision-making occurs at the top and there is a reluctance to embrace change, preferring instead to stick with tried and tested routines. |
| Club (also known as Power) | Zeus | Power is concentrated in the hands of one individual and radiates from the center. Networks and friendships define the decision-making process, which can happen quickly. However, the quality of decisions made will depend on the boss and the inner circle of influence. |
| Task | Athena | Power is derived from the expertise required to complete a task. Decision-making is more collaborative and based on merit. There are high degrees of adaptability and innovation, but this is countered by the expense associated with running such organizations, which often makes them short lived. |
| Existential (also known as People) | Dionysus | Exists to enable the individual to achieve their own goals. Employees have *lent* their skills and expertise to the organization and consequently, decision-making is devolved to the skilled professionals working within the organization. |

Source: adapted from ProvenModels (2018)

of organization may be unlikely, as it would need to be approved at committee level, which could challenge any change to the status quo.

In 2018, the National Health Service (NHS) was 70 years old. As the largest public sector employer in the UK with 1.64 million employees (Office for National Statistics 2018), it represents the perfect model of a role-based culture due to its hierarchical and bureaucratic nature. The tendency of bureaucratic organizations to form vertical structures or silos suggests that a playful workplace within the context of a role culture might feature competitive team games which pit one department against another. It is interesting to recall hospital inter-departmental ball games such as football, netball or rounders which were popular a few decades ago, when hospitals still had associated sports grounds and clubs. Collaborative working across departments within a role-based culture is naturally problematic but the recent trend towards multi-disciplinary team working gives some cause for celebration. In recent years, group singing in organized choirs, such as the NHS Choir, which is made up of multi-disciplinary staff from Lewisham and Greenwich NHS Trust in South-East London (Giddins 2018), represents a positive example of workplace playfulness. Singing in choirs offers numerous benefits, including improvements in self-confidence as well as enhancing posture and poise (Strange 2018). It can also promote social interaction and the confidence to perform in other contexts (ibid.), which offers further tangible benefits. In the case of the NHS Choir, profits raised from sales of a charity record which became the 'Christmas Number One' in the UK music charts in 2015, were passed to Mind, Carers UK and other smaller charities (Giddins 2018).

Playing with Lego$^{TM}$ has become increasingly popular within the world of business and research, through platforms such as Lego Serious Play. Lego allows stories and scenarios to be mapped-out or re-enacted, creating a learning environment which has been shown to remove hierarchical barriers, thereby enhancing communication and providing a shared learning experience for all (Tonkin 2016). Research has also shown that the collective building process generates heightened activity in the social areas of the brain (Gauntlett et al. 2011) and develops a range of positive attributes due to personal investment in the creative process (Norton et al. 2011).

## Club (also known as power) cultures

A strong departmental manager within an organization may have such strong leadership skills that the culture is more akin to the club culture. Power is held by the leader and those close to him/her (ProvenModels 2018). There are few rules or regulations and those with power make the decisions. A club culture is usually a strong culture, although its success is entirely dependent on the leader who holds the power. Those seeking to assume greater power within the organization, do so by getting close to the center (the leader). Ensuring the leader wins on the golf-course is a prime example of how playfulness might work in the club culture! A good leader in a club culture will nurture their staff and care for their wellbeing, using stories to paint a picture that is attractive, achievable, and exciting and which allows people to see how their work can fit into the organization (NHS Leadership

Academy 2013). The leader is responsible for championing learning and for driving skills development, using a broad range of experiences to enable people to develop their own potential. This might include learning from both success and failure (ibid.). In this context, play-based strategies involving simulation and role play can enhance skill development in a safe, supportive and non-threatening manner (Walsh 2016).

When using play as a means of exploration, humor can be a powerful tool for exerting social control as well as for promoting social engagement (Rogers 2016). For example, the popular television series *The Office* exemplified many aspects of workplace health and wellbeing through humorous caricatures that lampooned office politics (BBC 2018). The main character, David Brent, demonstrates the detrimental effects of poor leadership, failing to appreciate the impact of his own behavior and emotions on his colleagues (NHS Leadership Academy 2013). This television series has subsequently served as a rich training resource, demonstrating how the contrasting model of caring leadership can be achieved, along with its associated benefits (Nudd 2006).

## Task cultures

In a task culture, the task itself is the most important thing and power within the team varies according to the skills needed for each specific undertaking. Power may therefore transfer from one team member to another, according to how much they contribute to the task in hand. Task cultures revolve on team dynamics and, at their best, are both productive and creative (de Sousa Barbeta 2014). Any act of playfulness in this sort of culture needs to be task-related and best practice would demonstrate whole team involvement. Team members who do not have a role in achieving the set task, or who simply do not 'fit' with the group, can find themselves isolated from the rest of their work colleagues. Creative workplace environments seem to be particularly associated with task cultures. Play is manifest through organizational behaviors, providing a means of engagement that generates a positive climate which subsequently becomes part of the creative process itself (ibid.). In a workplace that actively promotes play as part of the daily routine, creating opportunities for workers to play computer games or to interact playfully with colleagues, results in a happy workforce that thrives on open communication. Within this climate, people are offered the time and space to be creative, and the sharing of ideas in a spirit of collaboration is actively encouraged (ibid.).

## People cultures

The fourth culture described by Handy, people culture, is an unusual culture and not found in many organizations (Businessballs 2017). Often depicted as 'a loose cluster or constellation of stars', people culture is focused on the individual worker, who is regarded as unique and superior to the environment in which they work (Businessballs 2017). With the drive to more accountability in the workplace, there is less and less likelihood of any one individual being able to operate in this manner, as the organizational structure exists to further the individual's own interests. Examples of people cultures include freelance workers, consultancies, architectural firms and universities, with the 'experts' benefiting from the 'power of their profession' (ibid.). Any playing in this culture would have to be an extension of the individual's wishes and wants.

It is possible to find aspects of all the four cultures identified by Handy within the overall role culture of an organization. Given this potential overlap, play and playfulness are evolving as key strategies within the field of Human Resources. Approaches to recruitment and training need to accommodate each different work culture within the organization. Many companies are now using games in the selection process for new employees (gamelearn 2018). When using games, fun is identified as a key component of the process, which can increase satisfaction when completing tasks and objectives, thus boosting self-esteem and revealing candidates' natural attributes (ibid.). Beyond selection, training and development are also utilizing games-based learning, which is being heralded as the 'present and future of e-learning' (ibid.).

The epitome of a positive, play-based culture is the LEGO Group. With its core values of 'Creativity, Imagination, Fun, Learning, Quality & Care' reflected in all aspects of its operation, the LEGO People Promise enables the execution of a business strategy designed to build and maintain the long-term health of the company – and its workers (Heryita n.d.). LEGO demonstrate that a company is built upon its culture and that this culture then becomes its heritage and an essential part of the business (ibid.). With play and playfulness increasingly becoming part of the culture of many workplaces, this also bodes well for life beyond work.

## Preparing for retirement and beyond

For many people, their working life will have been safe and healthy, rewarding the individual with a sense of self-worth and with opportunities for social functioning (TUC 2010). Retirement from the life of work is a phase which most workers generally look forward to but the transition can prove problematic for some people, invoking apprehension about the future including concerns about finances and self-identity (Fisher 2018). Retirement is therefore also a key area for public health activity (Public Health England 2016).

There is a plethora of advice for those approaching retirement, although most of this is about assuring financial security, particularly in relation to pensions, pension pots and personal savings. However, a focus on financial planning denies the need for emotional guidance through the transition to life after retirement. Stopping work represents a major lifestyle change which may be accompanied by parallel upheavals such as downsizing the home or geographical relocation. There may be anxieties about personal relationships and the impact of a new non-work regime. There are plenty of jokes about male partners, the traditional breadwinners, intruding or interfering in the protected domain of the other partner (usually female) after retirement. 'Retired Husband Syndrome' has been shown to cause stress and depression in spouses which increases year on year following the husband's retirement (Lambert 2014).

It is odd to say that retirement comes as a surprise, given that most workers have a clear idea (even a countdown) of when they plan to stop work, but neither employees nor their employers really consider how to prepare for what may be several decades of not working. Consideration of the potential benefits of play, and active planning to include play and playfulness into the lives of retired people, would be a way of assuring emotional preparedness.

The transition period between working life and retired life is a crucial phase that is often associated with anxiety and depression, even when it has been eagerly antici-pated and planned for (Fisher 2018). The loss of identity, routine, and purpose has been equated to the grieving process, which can be summarized as follows:

- *Denial*: 'Oh No, Not ME, I can't be retirement age, can I?'
- *Anger*: 'They forced me out, I hate retirement, my job was so wonderful … not.'
- *Depression*: 'What do I do all day? Couch potato, here I come …'
- *Acceptance*: 'Hmmm, not so bad, found purpose, feel great, life is so good!'

*(Fisher 2018)*

Reaching a point of acceptance will invariably involve advance-planning. Introdu-cing elements of play and playfulness prior to retirement can help to alleviate potential fears, particularly in relation to the effective and productive use of time, concepts which have prevailed during the years of employment (MensLine Australia 2018). Continuity Theory suggests that 'in making adaptive choices, middle-aged and older adults attempt to preserve and maintain existing internal and external structures…tied to their past experiences of themselves and their social world. Continuity is thus a grand adaptive strategy that is promoted by both individual preference and social approval' (Atchley 1989: 183). Payson (2019) suggests that, according to continuity theory, an individual's personality, behaviors and preferences are stable and will remain similar into older age. Therefore, if the retiree has experienced play and playfulness in their work culture it would be second nature to carry a playful disposition into retired life and to expand on it accordingly. Retirement offers opportunities to devote more time to established hobbies and interests while also raising the possibility of taking-on something new. According to Frey Waxman (2003: 83) 'courageously plunging into new experiences, elderly deep players often gain new insights and attain self-accep-tance for their bravery – as well as simply having more fun'.

Older age is often seen as a time of 'passivity, decline and increasing isolation' (Frey Waxman 2003: 79) but this is rapidly being challenged. The traditional retirement age is increasing as people live longer, and in the UK it is estimated that more than one million people aged over 65 years of age are still in some form of employment (Black 2016). This is leading to an emphasis on utilizing the latter years of working life to prepare for retirement, applying this time to 'cultivate the habit of living more in the present, with intentionality and passion' (Frey-Waxman 2003: 79).

Elders are particularly suited to involvement in deep play, and engagement with nature offers the 'time and space for absorption that moves the player beyond the intentionality of the setting' (Frey Waxman 2003: 81). Engaging with nature can include a range of differing physical activities at a time when reduced stamina and declining balance may be causing difficulties. Nature-based group walks are associated with significantly reduced depressive states and perceived stress, while conversely promoting greater positive mental wellbeing (Lawson 2015). Nature also exemplifies the individuality of deep play, as noted by Frey Waxman (2003: 82) who explains that 'the simple activities of examining patterns of shells in a small space at the shore or observing the movements of birds in mountain forests are other forms of deep play for me'. The significance of play in nature and its associated health benefits are discussed more fully in chapters 3 and 12.

Retirement is an opportunity to try-out a range of less physically demanding activities which may previously have been overlooked (Frey Waxman 2003). As Public Health England (2016) suggest, in Figure 10.1, it is never too late to be physically active and 'any physical activity is better than none'. Adaptations to sporting activities, such as walking football or walking netball, have become popular pastimes for people over the age of 50 years of age, with the Walking Football Association (2018) reporting that many tournaments are now exclusively being run for the over-60s age group. Teams usually comprise five to six players and matches are played on 3G artificial grass pitches, thus minimizing the risk of pain, injury and discomfort (ibid.).

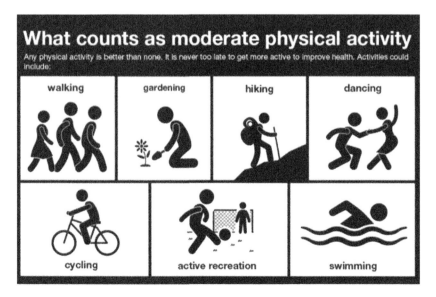

FIGURE 10.1 Identifying what counts as physical activity.
Source: Public Health England (2016)

Play fulfils important cultural and biological functions that are embedded in society (Huizinga 1949) and activities which attract the attention of the community provide opportunities for new social engagement (Frey Waxman 2003). Since the global financial crisis of 2007 and the subsequent period of austerity, there have been abundant opportunities for the recently retired person to act in a voluntary capacity in what were previously paid positions, typically in meet-and-greet, educational and caring roles. Some of these opportunities involve taking-on a playful persona. Many museums, gardens and historical sites, for example, have informed greeters who dress-up to recount amusing anecdotes about the location. Time is a precious commodity and 'giving to others' of one's own time accords a sense of purpose and personal fulfilment while boosting self-esteem, as well as serving the wider community and creating communication networks (Foresight Mental Capital and Wellbeing Project 2008).

The University of the Third Age (commonly referred to as U3A) aims to educate and stimulate those 'mainly retired members of the community – those in their third "age" of life' (U3A Sources 2018). As a lifelong learning movement which started in 1982, U3A now works with over 1000 'member learning cooperative charities and organizations in the United Kingdom' (U3A 2018: 4). Although an international movement, U3A mainly provides activities locally including lectures and workshops, many of which are quite light-hearted and playful. Built on the concept of 'skill sharing, mutuality and inclusion' and peer-to-peer learning (ibid.: 4), participants are entertained and amused, not just educated. Play and playfulness can extend friendships beyond the original U3A activities. For example, 'members spoke of giving exhibitions or playing music or playing pétanque [a game similar to boules] outside of the U3A, and finding groups of members who would come and support them at external events' (ibid.: 14). U3A (ibid.: 19) counters the traditional 'deficit and dependency approach to ageing [offering] … an alternative ageing experience, which is built on shared learning, skill sharing and volunteering'.

The inclusion of play as a fundamental part of life as a retired person has advantages for emotional, mental and physical health. Leading a long and healthy life as a retired person is an aspiration for all of us and embracing play and playfulness in all its diverse and adaptive forms can help us to achieve this.

## Conclusion

Marmot (2010: 20) stated that 'work is good – and unemployment bad – for physical and mental health, but the quality of work matters' (ibid.: 20). Few people would disagree with the premise that workplace environments should be kind and caring places that are inclusive and encourage collaborative working. Workers should be active, energetic and creative, and play provides the perfect vehicle to facilitate this. Play and playfulness are known for their nurturing, restorative and non-threatening qualities, offering much to the embodiment of good work. A happy and engaged workforce is mutually beneficial to the employee and employer alike, as noted by the Greek philosopher Aristotle (cited in TUC 2010) who stated that 'pleasure in the job puts perfection in the work'. A playful workplace is also favourable to retirement, as supported by continuity theory. behaviors and dispositions built up over a lifetime of employment can be deployed through volunteering, skill sharing or just by enjoying life and having fun. For some, the concept of a working life never ends, as noted by Hugh Hefner, who stated: 'I have no plans to retire. It's the perfect combination of work and play that keeps you young. If I quit work, it would be the beginning of the end for me' (BrainyQuote 2018).

## References

Atchley, R. (1989) A Continuity Theory of Normal Aging, *The Gerontologist*, 29(2): 183–190.

BBC (2018) The Office, retrieved from www.bbc.co.uk/programmes/p0045rb0 (accessed 15 August 2018).

Black, C. (2016) Keeping the Workforce Healthy, in All Party Parliamentary Group and the Health Foundation (ed.), *A Healthier Life for All: The Case for Cross-government Action*, 30–31, London: The Health Foundation.

Bradshaw, C. (2013) People Achieve More by Combining Work and Play, retrieved from www.thirdsector.co.uk/people-achieve-combining-work-play/finance/article/1180335 (accessed 9 July 2018).

BrainyQuote (2018) Hugh Hefner Quotes, retrieved from www.brainyquote.com/authors/hugh_hefner (accessed 16 August 2018).

Businessballs (2017) Organisational Culture, retrieved from www.businessballs.com/organisational-culture/types-of-organisational-culture-4051 (accessed 24 July 2018).

Csikszentmihalyi, M. (2009) *Creativity: Flow and the Psychology of Discovery and Invention*, New York: Harper Perennial.

Department for Work and Pensions and Department of Health (2016) *Improving Lives the Work, Health and Disability Green Paper*, London: Department for Work and Pensions and Department of Health.

De Sousa Barbeta, A. (2014) The Importance of Recognising Playfulness to Develop Creativity: The Case of Blip Web Engineers, dissertation, University of Porto, Portugal.

Everett, A. (2011) Benefits and Challenges of Fun in the Workplace, *Library Leadership and Management*, 25(1): 1–10.

Fisher, W. (2018) Retirement Anxiety Hurts … But it Doesn't Have To. It's Time to LIVE Life!, retrieved from www.retirement-online.com/after-retirement-anxiety-and-depression.html (accessed 5 August 2018).

Foresight Mental Capital and Wellbeing Project (2008) *Final Project Report*, London: Government Office for Science.

Frey Waxman, B. (2003) Retiring into Intensity, Experiencing Deep Play, in N. Bauer-Maglin and A. Radosh (eds), *Women Confronting Retirement: A Non-traditional Guide*: 79–88, New Brunswick, NJ: Rutgers University Press.

gamelearn (2018) The Game as the New Strategy in Human Resources, retrieved from www.game-learn.com/game-new-strategy-human-resources (accessed 16 August 2018).

Gauntlett, D., Ackermann, E., Whitebread, D., Wolbers, T. and Weckstrom, C. (2011) *The Future of Play: Defining the Role and Value of Play in the 21st Century*, Billund: LEGO Institute.

Giddins, K. (2018) Dazzling Doctors: Who Are the NHS Choir, Who Is Choirmaster Dr Katie Rogerson and When Did They Have a Christmas Number One?, retrieved from www.thesun.co.uk/tvandshowbiz/6341165/nhs-choir-christmas-number-one-album (accessed 2 August 2018).

Handy, C. (1978) *Gods of Management: The Changing Work of Organizations*, Oxford: Oxford University Press.

Heryita, R. (n.d.) A Great Company Culture Example: LEGO, retrieved from https://inside.6q.io/company-culture-example-lego (accessed 16 August 2018).

Huizinga, J. (1949) *Homo Ludens*, London: Taylor & Francis.

Institute of Health Equality (2018) Create Fair Employment and Good Work for All, retrieved from www.instituteofhealthequity.org/resources-reports/create-fair-employment-and-good-work-for-all- (accessed 9 July 2018).

Lambert, V. (2014) Retired Husband Syndrome – Why Wives Get Depressed When Their Other Halves Stop Working, *The Telegraph*, 22 August, retrieved from www.telegraph.co.uk/women/womens-life/11048659/Retired-husband-syndrome-why-wives-get-dep ressed-when-their-other-halves-stop-working.html (accessed 15 August 2018).

Lawson, K. (2015) Woodland Walks and your 'Elf', retrieved from www.nationalelfservice.net/treatment/exercise/woodland-walks-and-your-elf (accessed 15 August 2018).

Local Government Association (2018) Marmot Review Report – 'Fair Society, Healthy Lives, retrieved from www.local.gov.uk/marmot-review-report-fair-society-healthy-lives (accessed 23 July 2018).

Marmot, M. (2010) Fair Society, Healthy Lives: The Marmot Review Executive Summary, retrieved from www.instituteofhealthequity.org/resources-reports/fair-society-healthy-li ves-the-marmot-review/fair-society-healthy-lives-exec-summary-pdf.pdf (accessed 9 July 2018).

MensLine Australia (2018) Adjusting to Retirement, retrieved from https://mensline.org.au/tips-and-tools/adjusting-to-retirement (accessed 5 August 2018).

Minds for Business (2017) Playing Up the Benefits of Play at Work, retrieved from www.psychologicalscience.org/news/minds-business/playing-up-the-benefits-of-play-at-work.html (accessed 9 July 2018).

NHS Leadership Academy (2013) *Healthcare Leadership Model: The Nine Dimensions of Leadership behaviour*, Leeds: NHS Leadership Academy.

Norton, M. I., Mochon, D. and Ariely, D. (2011) The IKEA Effect: When Labor Leads to Love, *Journal of Consumer Psychology*, 22(3): 453–460.

Nudd, T. (2006) David Brent Shows Microsoft How it's Done, retrieved from www.adweek.com/creativity/david-brent-shows-microsoft-how-it-s-done-18462 (accessed 15 August 2018).

Office for National Statistics (2018) Public Sector Employment, UK: March 2018, Online. HTTP:<www.ons.gov.uk/employmentandlabourmarket/peopleinwork/publicsectorp ersonnel/bulletins/publicsectoremployment/march2018#employment-in-public-adminis tration-and-the-national-health-service-rises (accessed 15 August 2018).

Payson, M. (2019) Biological and Social Theories of Aging, in H. Lohman, S. Byers-Connon and L. Padilla (eds), *Occupational Therapy with Elders: Strategies for the COTA*, 4th edition, Oxford: Elsevier.

Pflug, K. and Jara, J. (2014) Workplace Fun and Games Motivate Employees, *Workspan*, December: 50–54.

ProvenModels (2018) Gods of Management, retrieved from www.provenmodels.com/8/gods-of-management/charles-b.-handy (accessed 24 July 2018).

Public Health England (2016) Guidance: Health Matters: Getting Every Adult Active Every Day, retrieved from www.gov.uk/government/publications/health-matters-getting-e very-adult-active-every-day/health-matters-getting-every-adult-active-every-day (acces sed 13 November 2017).

Public Health England (2018) The Importance of Health and Work, retrieved from www.gov.uk/government/publications/health-and-work-infographics/the-importance-of-hea lth-and-work (accessed 12 July 2018).

Rogers, T. (2016) It's Often Forgotten: Humour Is a Brilliant Way of Mastering Classroom Management, retrieved from www.tes.com/news/school-news/breaking-views/its-of ten-forgotten-humour-a-brilliant-way-mastering-classroom (accessed 7 October 2016).

Strange, C. (2018) In Search of Harmony, *Breath*, 9: 46–47.

Taylor, M. (2017) Good Work: The Taylor Review of Modern Working Practices, retrieved from https://assets.publishing.service.gov.uk/government/uploads/system/uploads/attachm ent_data/file/627671/good-work-taylor-review-modern-working-practices-rg.pdf (accessed 27 August 2018).

Taylor, P. (2016) How Our Organisations Can Stifle Community Creativity, retrieved from https://medium.com/@PaulBromford/how-our-organisations-can-stifle-community-crea tivity-84d86d1e06d4 (accessed 23 July 2018).

Tonkin, A. (2016) Playful Design, in A. Tonkin, and J. Whitaker (eds), *Play in Healthcare for Adults: Using Play to Promote Health and Wellbeing Across the Adult Lifespan*, 212–225, Abingdon: Routledge.

TUC (2010) *In Sickness and in Health? Good Work – and How to Achieve it*, London: TUC.

U3A (2018) *Learning Not Lonely: Living Life, Expanding Horizons Challenging Conventions*, London: The Third Age Trust.

U3A Sources (2018) U3A and 'the 5 Ways to Wellbeing', *U3A Sources*, 26 January, retrieved from https://sources.u3a.org.uk/2018/01/26/u3a-and-the-5-ways-to-wellbeing (accessed 16 August 2018).

University of Portsmouth (2013) Black Humour Bonds Police and Ambulance Crews, retrieved from http://uopnews.port.ac.uk/2013/02/07/black-humour-bonds-police-a nd-ambulance-crews (accessed 14 August 2018).

Van Vleet, M. and FeeneyB. (2015) Play Behavior and Playfulness in Adulthood, *Social and Personality Psychology Compass*, 9(11): 630–643.

Walking Football Association (2018) What Is Walking Football?, retrieved from https:// thewfa.co.uk (accessed 15 August 2018).

Walsh, A. (2016) Think Play Is for Nurseries, Not Universities? Think Again, retrieved from www.theguardian.com/higher-education-network/2016/sep/01/think-play-is-for-nurser ies-not-universities-think-again (accessed 1 September 2016).

# 11

# PLAYING IN A DIGITAL WORLD

*Alison Tonkin*

## Introduction

Almost 100 years ago, Winslow (1920) identified three distinct phases of public health history. Firstly, acknowledgement of sanitation as a causative factor in the spread of disease and plague. Secondly, the bacteriological phase which saw the emergence of immunization and vaccination; and thirdly, the role of education and the 'hygienic guidance of the individual living machine' (ibid.: 29). Public health also has a rich recent history, and although the past century has seen many developments in thinking and practice, a fourth phase of public health has now emerged – the era of digital public health.

According to Black and Dixon (2017), digital public health is about 'a reimaging of public health using … new ways of working, blending established public health wisdom with new digital concepts and tools'. Play and playfulness have been embraced as key components of many public health interventions and activities, designed to engage both the general population and professionals at individual and societal levels in this new vision of public health. While acknowledging widespread concern about the infiltration of digital media into all aspects of modern life (Bartlett 2018), this chapter focuses on how ludic creativity is being assimilated into a wide range of public health initiatives. This is the case both knowingly with foresight and planning, as in the case of the National Elf Service (2018), but also accidentally, as demonstrated by the popularity of Pokémon GO and the Metro Trains Melbourne Dumb Ways to Die campaign, both of which have been recognized as two of the most effective public health innovations in recent years (Hinsliff 2016; Jardine 2017).

## Defining digital public health

Public Health England (2017) introduce the context of digital public health in relation to how technology has changed and now influences how we 'live, interact, learn, play and work'. This suggests new possibilities for engaging and interacting with people on a far wider scale that is both 'agile' and timely, providing flexible services which are responsive to the needs of individuals and communities in an equitable and accessible manner (ibid.). The United Kingdom is seen as a world leader in digital transformation and was ranked first by the United Nations in 2016 for e-government and e-participation linked to participatory decision-making (United Nations 2018). The UK is recognized as leading the drive towards digital health and is keen to share its expertise oversees (UK Government 2016). Public Health England (PHE), as an executive agency of the Department of Health and Social Care in the UK, has developed a digital strategy that aims to 'make best use of technology to protect and promote health and reduce inequalities' (Public Health England 2017).

The Oxford English Dictionary (2018a), defines technology as 'the application of scientific knowledge for practical purposes' and digital as 'involving or relating to the use of computer technology' (Oxford English Dictionary 2018b). Digital technology encompasses 'social, mobile, analytics and cloud technologies [which] have been joined by advances in automation and sensors, 3-D printing, robotics, wearables, and technology… including machine learning, augmented reality and artificial intelligence' (Black and Dixon 2017).

The World Health Organization (2016: viii) defines digital health as: 'The use of digital, mobile and wireless technologies to support the achievement of health objectives. Digital health describes the general use of information and communications technologies (ICT) for health and is inclusive of both mHealth and eHealth' (ibid.).

Digital public health represents an extension of the medical and healthcare objectives of digital health to provide a broader, holistic overview of health that incorporates, yet goes beyond, the needs of the individual to address community health issues at local, national and international levels. Public Health England (2017) identifies a reduction in health inequalities as one of the key aims of their digital public health strategy. While 77 per cent of people in the UK have basic digital skills, 12.6 million adults remain digitally illiterate (Open Forum Events 2018). If public health is to be truly inclusive of all members of society, including citizens and public health professionals, there is a need for further innovation and creativity. However, 'established public health wisdom' is not easily overcome: Black (2016) comments:

> I am reminded of the old joke 'drink coffee and do stupid things faster'. Doing the same old stuff digitally misses the point – digital tools and ways of working offer a chance to transform what we do and how we do it.

Play is taking a leading role in this digital transformation.

## Playing with public health

The application of play, and particularly game play, is providing a paradigm for promoting learning, improving skills and changing behavior (Pflug and Jara 2014) for individuals, communities and the public health professionals who serve them.

This is exemplified by the emergence of the Games for Health Journal, a relatively new periodical that provides peer-reviewed articles that are 'dedicated to advancing the impact of game research, technologies, and applications on human health and well-being' (see www.liebertpub.com/g4h). The gamification of healthcare, using game elements for non-gaming purposes, uses behavioral science and psychology to improve the motivation of behavior change, by presenting healthful activities as fun as opposed to hard work (Warner 2016). However, Sailer et al. (2017) suggest that gamification tends to be seen as a 'generic construct', which fails to acknowledge that differing game design elements elicit widely varying applications and can therefore address a range of 'basic psychological needs'. They go on to provide a number of examples, stating: 'Our results show that badges, leader boards, and performance graphs positively affect competence need satisfaction, as well as perceived task meaningfulness, while avatars, meaningful stories, and teammates affect experiences of social relatedness'. Table 11.1 explores a range of game design elements and offers examples of how each has been applied in public health practice.

The two main methodological approaches commonly associated with public health are *serious games* and *gamification*, which have many similarities in how they motivate the participant. Pappas (2017) has identified four common benefits linked to eLearning situations which can also be applied to public health activities and interventions:

1.  Motivation of online learners.
2.  Putting knowledge into practice.
3.  Sparking friendly competition.
4.  Facilitating mistake-driven learning.

### Motivation of online learners

For those who lack the intrinsic motivation to participate in health-promoting activities, both serious games and gamification use *nudges* to encourage users to actively take part in the activity. Incentives such as earning badges, extra points and rewards are examples of this kind of positive reinforcement (Pappas 2017). SuperBetter is a positive psychology game linked to Cognitive Behavior Therapy (CBT). It allows players to advance through different levels by earning points (Fleming et al. 2017), building-up psychological resilience through narrative and social support (Johnson et al. 2016). SuperBetter also uses an approach known as *snacktivity* whereby healthy activities lasting just a few minutes are played frequently over the course of a day or a longer period. As a mental health tool, this game has shown significant reductions in depression and anxiety by those who completed 10 minutes of activities each day over a 30-day period, although the attrition rate was also noticeably high (Fleming et al. 2017).

**TABLE 11.1** Play methodologies linked to applications in public health.

| Game design elements | Description | Applied examples |
|---|---|---|
| *Gamification* | Elements of games that are used outside the traditional concept of games (Fleming et al. 2017). Often linked to traditional eLearning activities, gamification uses games mechanics to provide incentives that promote active engagement by the user (Pappas 2017). | Zombies, Run! is a mobile application that encourages participants to walk, jog or run while listening to music and a narrative through headphones. As the game proceeds, zombies chase the participant, encouraging them run to faster, as well as automatically picking-up supplies such as virtual medicines, clothing and zombie killing equipment to enable survival in a Zombie apocalypse (see https://zombiesrungame.com). |
| *Serious Games* | Computerized games that are used for serious purposes (Fleming et al. 2017). Serious games will follow a typical games structure but integrate some elements of skill-based learning as part of the process. According to Pappas (2017) 'serious games are fun, entertaining, and interactive' but, unlike gamification, 'serious games can exist independently'. However, they should not be used as a stand-alone approach to eLearning but can be used as a complement to other leaning activities (Pappas 2017). | When used as a means of simulation, Serious Games can provide a low-cost alternative to traditional simulation methodologies, using a simple CD-Rom or DVD. They can also be used to recreate complex situations which cannot be replicated in real life (see http://publichealthgames.com). The School of Health Promotion at the University of Illinois at Chicago uses this approach to provide training for public health officials and emergency responders using simulation that is 'fun and engaging'. This includes Anthrax Simulation, which replicates a potential bioterrorism attack in Chicago, USA. The simulation is designed to train 'thousands of people to dispense mass amounts of drugs in the wake of a large-scale anthrax attack'. |
| *Game theory* | A branch of applied mathematics that can be used to problem-solve contemporary issues, providing solutions to public health issues (Malhotra 2012). Game play is interdependent which means each player must consider other participant responses prior to generating their own (ibid.). | Game Theory is particularly effective for modelling community health interventions, particularly when incentives for individuals may be detrimental to the beneficial outcomes of a community. Schüller, Stanková and Thuijsman (2017) provide a 'simple game-theoretical model of pollution control, where each country is in control of its own pollution, while the environmental effects of policies do not stop at country borders'. The game can be used to explore incentives that promote environmentally friendly policies. |

| Game design elements | Description | Applied examples |
| --- | --- | --- |
| Intergenerational Games (IGG) | The use of digital games to provide opportunities for differing generations to engage and interact with one another through digital platforms (Digital Unite 2018). Digital learning can be linked to other activities, in this instance games that can be played across the generations. | Wii video games consoles can play a variety of popular games such as Monopoly, Scrabble and Connect 4 which can be used to engage younger and older generations, mitigating the potential impact of social isolation and loneliness. Young people can teach older people how to use gaming consoles for interactive gaming, which can be played through computers or remotely online over the internet (Digital Unite 2018). |

## Putting knowledge into practice

Real-life situations can be linked to fictional characters, enabling players to face challenges through simulation and the re-creation of challenging or complex situations. This approach enables players to experiment with differing skills and problem-solving strategies that might be used in real-life situations (Pappas 2017). For example, the Secret of Seven Stones (SSS) is an intergenerational video game designed to provide sexual health communication skills training for young people aged 11–14 years and their parents in the home environment. As a means of addressing public health issues linked to sexual behavior (i.e. reducing risk related behavior; delaying the initiation of sexual relationships; and maintaining healthy 'friendships') this IGG provides an 'inclusive and shared experience for parents and youth to provide a common meeting ground for sexual health discussion' (Pravanta et al. 2018: 188).

## Sparking friendly competition

The use of competitive 'leader boards' provides additional motivation and a means of assessing how well people are engaging with an activity. However, not everyone enjoys the concept of leader boards and for some, this can detract from the gaming experience. Alternatives such as 'certificates or unlockable objects' also inspire competitiveness, but on a more personal level (Pappas 2017). Fitbit League enables users of Fitbit (a wearable physical activity tracker) to be ranked according to their individual activity times and to compete with one another around the world (see www.facebook.com/pg/fitbitleague). Communities of users can also interact with one another through Facebook, with a recent post stating that the Fitbit League is 'an online fitness league and a playground for active people', with the strap line exemplifying the social cohesion derived from exercising as a group: – 'Fitbit League – Together We Move' (Fitbit League 2017).

## Facilitating mistake-driven learning

Van Rijswijk (cited van Gool 2016) states that 'people are intrinsically motivated to play … [and] in a gamified setting, they can experiment and make mistakes in a secure environment'. Serious games and gamification use immediate feedback mechanisms which identify things that need improvement or activities that have gone well. This also allows trainers to identify where additional resources or support may be needed. Pappas (2017) identifies this as an opportunity to 'see the outcome and repercussions of their behaviors before they enter the real world. Every mistake online learners make is a chance to improve and reflect on their cognitions'. The International Journal of Public Health (2011) describes a variety of such games linked to public health education, including the Great Flu (see www.thegreatflu.com). Developed by the Erasmus MC University Medical Center in Rotterdam, participants 'choose the virus, choose the response, manage the budget, monitor infections and deaths' (ibid.). With different viruses having differing degrees of difficulty in terms of game play, the cause-and-effect nature of decision-making allows players to learn when things go wrong and to find alternative ways of winning the game.

The remainder of this chapter will examine in more detail three differing aspects of digital public health which have play and playfulness at their core.

## Sharing evidence among public health professionals

One of the major functions of public health is the collection, collation, analysis and dissemination of health-related data. Black and Dixon (2017) state: 'digital is about generating and using new kinds of data properly; it is about an open, and faster culture; and it is about learning by doing'. For any professional, it becomes increasingly difficult to keep up with the plethora of evidence from relevant and reliable sources (Tomlin and Badenoch 2015). Many practitioners also have difficulty 'finding, using and understanding', as well as appraising, evidence-based research which means that available innovations and evidence are not necessarily being applied to practice (ibid.). Tomlin and Badenoch (ibid.) conclude that, in this digital era, 'blogs and social media are essential tools that can help all health and social care professionals find, use and discuss relevant evidence' and go on to advocate 'blogging and tweeting as an excellent way to keep their knowledge current'.

In 2011, Tomlin and Badenoch (2015) started the National Elf Service, which exploits 'an unhealthy interest in puns' and uses animation to disseminate research-based evidence in an accessible and humorous manner. The National Elf Service provides an excellent example of how ludic creativity has been used as part of a 'new digital tool' to disseminate 'useful' evidence-based research which can be utilized by a multitude of specialist and non-specialist parties from a range of disciplines and perspectives (see Figure 11.1).

Each elf represents a topic area such as the Social Care Elf or the Dental Elf. The original Mental Elf responds to the proliferation of papers in the field of mental

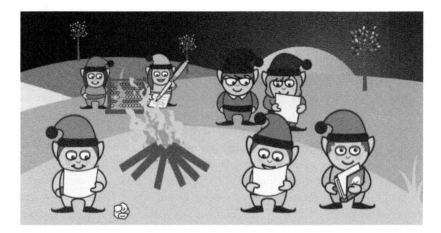

**FIGURE 11.1** Elves gathered around the campfire discussing evidence-based research.
Source: National Elf Service (2018); reproduced by kind permission of André Tomlin,
National Elf Service

health which would need to be read each day just to keep up to date with the
published research. This has risen from three papers per day in 1973 to a total
of 249 per day in 2013, resulting in the following comment from Tomlin and
Badenoch (2015): 'reading 249 papers a day is too much even for some elves
(mentioning no names). Evidence-based blogs of the research just make sense!'
The National Elf Service addresses this daily overload through 'a community of
research-savvy bloggers' who share and discuss the latest evidence around the
elf community campfire. There are now 11 elves along the 'woodland path',
each hosting blogs from over 100 diverse bloggers who make up the 'woodland
clan'. These include 'professors and journal editors writing blogs … service
users and carers, researchers, doctors, nurses, students, librarians and a broad
spectrum of health and social care professionals', from the global community,
with under half coming from Australasia, Canada, United States, Middle east
and Europe (National Elf Service 2018). The original Mental Elf is now one of
a community of 'Elf Professors' who each lead discussions in a different topic
area, such as social care, commissioning, stroke, the child, musculoskeletal,
learning disabilities and dental as well as three other areas covering diabetes,
education and lifestyle.

The imagery of a community of woodland elves chatting with one another around a
campfire is an engaging and inviting conceptual framework. It puts users at ease when
accessing technical and often complex information, as demonstrated in the two-minute
promotional video (National Elf Service 2018). The use of imagery is an important
feature of the website and the Mental Elf has been acclaimed for the creativity and
sensitivity of its blogs and the use of images as an interesting alternative to the more
usual representation of mental health issues (Chapman 2017).

As Cochrane UK's 'knowledge broker', Chapman (2017), writing for Evidently Cochrane, which aims to make complex evidence contained within the Cochrane Library's collection of systematic reviews easily accessible, humorously explores how the use of stock images to portray various health related content can actually make the reader question the content and consequently dilutes the validity of the message. The role of engagement and communication in the digital age has become big business and it is widely recognized that people connect with images that are both salient and authentic. This is exemplified in relation to issues such as sexual health, as covered during Evidently Cochrane's recent Twitter campaign #TheProblemWithSex.

## Pokémon GO – a global public health phenomenon

On 6 July 2016, Pokémon GO was released by Niantic when they turned the original Pokémon trading card game launched in 1995 into a mobile gaming app that is free to download and to play on handheld devices such as smartphones and tablets. Within the first eight weeks, the game was downloaded over 500 million times (Watanabe et al. 2017) and had more active users than Twitter (Knight 2016). Pokémon Go appeals to people across the age-range and from all walks of life, as shown when the Norwegian Prime Minister, Erna Solberg, was 'caught' playing Pokémon GO prior to meeting with Donald Trump in the White House (Zeroghan 2018).

Pokémon, which stands for *pocket monsters*, are 'creatures of all shapes and sizes who live in the wild or alongside humans…[who] are raised and commanded by their trainers' (Pokémon Company International 2018). The Pokémon 'family' of products includes video games (by Nintendo), the original trading card game, animated TV series and films, as well as toys in a variety of formats. One of the strengths of the game since its inception has been an emphasis on 'good sportsmanship and a respect for other players' (ibid.) and this is reflected in Pokémon GO, which has its own etiquette code that encourages social cohesion and consideration for other players (St Ive 2016).

Pokémon GO has a rallying call to 'Get up and go … Catch Pokémon in the real world', and the promotional trailer states: 'The world of Pokémon is all around you – go explore, go discover, go collect' (see www.pokemongo.com). The game uses augmented reality to create 'immersive gaming experiences that utilize your actual surroundings … allowing users to catch virtual Pokémon who are hidden throughout a map of the real world' (Augment 2018). Players need to search for, catch, and train Pokémon while collecting objects that allow differing facets of the game to be played. These include 'eggs' which contain versions of Pokémon waiting to hatch – and to hatch an egg, you need to walk 2, 5, 7 or 10 kilometers. Players progress through the game by leaving their homes or workplaces to go outdoors and walk (Watanabe et al. 2017). Habitual behavior, such as an inactive, sedentary lifestyle, has traditionally resisted change by conventional means (Knight 2016), but Pokémon GO has shown that having fun is itself a motivating factor, irrespective of the health-related benefits (Baranowski 2016).

Much of the anecdotal evidence of the benefits associated with playing Pokémon GO is linked to the promotion of physical activity (Hinsliff 2016; Watanabe et al. 2017). van Rijswijk (cited van Gool 2016) who is the chairman of the Games for Health Europe Foundation, describes Pokémon GO as a 'textbook example of gamification for health' due to its playful contribution to players fitness, inviting them to have fun while increasing activity levels. Pleasurable experiences activate the brain reward pathways which in turn motivates the player to repeat the rewarding behavior (Perry et al. 2000). Chapter 2 elaborates on how play triggers this reward mechanism. Dopamine neurons are known to mediate behavior and game developers refer to the concept of *dopamine squirters*, which provide small, frequent doses of dopamine as a means of positive reinforcement, keeping the reward pathways operating and game play consistently pleasurable and self-reinforcing (Washington 2012). A common misconception by health gamification designers is that physical fitness must be the primary aim of the game. van Rijswijk suggests that, in fact, the opposite is true: the fun element of the game should be the starting point, which is why Pokémon GO has been so successful (van Gool 2016).

Health is a holistic concept and engagement with one aspect of health is likely to have a knock-on effect on other aspects (Whitaker and Tonkin 2016). In addition to promoting physical activity, playing Pokémon GO has been associated with improvements in the mental health of players (Knight 2016). Watanabe et al. (2017) researched the impact of playing Pokémon Go on the psychological distress levels of 3,195 full-time workers in Japan, through the completion of self-report questionnaires. Results showed a significant reduction in psychological distress in those who played the game compared with those who did not, and Watanabe concluded that 'the game could have positive effects on the mental health of the adult working population' (ibid.: 1). Pokémon Go has also been shown to help people with autism, depression and social withdrawal (Watanabe et al. 2017) due to the promotion of socialization and the need for players to work together (St Ive 2016).

The role of the community in improving health and wellbeing has been widely recognized, particularly in relation to combatting social isolation (Buck and Wenzel, 2018). Pokémon Go communities come together at a local level to play features of the game that demand collaboration with other players. Pokémon Go prides itself on promoting social cohesion and a peaceful gaming platform that appeals to children and adults alike (St Ive 2016). It is often serviced by the gaming app Discord (Discord n.d.) and run by moderators from the Discord community who might not ordinarily connect with other players in the 'real world'. The contribution to public health made by Pokémon Go is captured by Sebastian Yuen, a paediatrician, who tweeted, 'I think @PokémonGoApp is an awesome example of how tech can help public health. It encourages exercise, builds real life communities and has great game mechanics and very frequent updates to max engagement MUCH better than #Fitbit!' (Yuen 2018).

Hinsliff (2016) recognizes that the acceptance of new technology needs to pass through three stages, the final stage of which represents a 'moral panic' in terms of what the technology reveals about human nature. In the case of Pokémon Go, 'people have done dumb and risky things while playing' but if you replace 'playing Pokémon Go with almost any activity … that sentence remains true' (ibid.). The following example is a case in point.

## Playful engagement with accident prevention

Public health aims to 'provide the maximum benefit for the largest number of people' (World Health Organization 2018) and this demands novel ways to ensure public health messages are accessible and that they are relevant to the intended audience. Reducing health inequalities is a prerequisite of any public health measure: adults from areas of deprivation are twice as likely to be hospitalized, and twice as likely to die from unintentional injury, as those from less deprived areas (RoSPA 2013). RoSPA (www.rospa.com) identifies accidents as the biggest threat to families throughout the lifespan, noting that 14,000 people a year die in the UK due to accidents. RoSPA (2018) have identified accident prevention as the number one priority for public health, stating that the prevention of accidental injury is relatively easy to deliver, at relatively low cost, but the outcomes are high impact. In 2012, Metro Trains Melbourne ran a Public Service Announcement (PSA) that became a global phenomenon, with the video going viral on YouTube and the associated song, performed by Tangerine Kitty, reaching number 10 on the iTunes chart within days of its release (Dumb Ways to Die 2018a). Jardine (2017) describes the key characteristics of the campaign, noting how it 'tapped into two elements that are loved almost universally: catchy music and cute cartoon characters. Add some really black humor into the mix and you get the beginnings of a cult classic.'

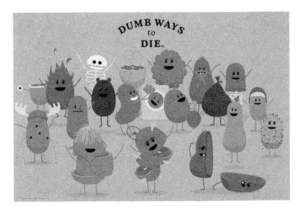

**FIGURE 11.2** The original cast representing 'dumb ways to die'.
Source: reproduced by kind permission of Dean Mendes, Metro Trains Melbourne Pty Ltd

The campaign matched lyrics which named a variety of 'dumb ways to die' to cartoon characters who would 'graphically meet their fate in various sick ways' (Jardine 2017). It highlighted a range of potentially fatal accidents, including 'eat medicine that's out of date … get your toast out with a fork … eat a two-week-old unrefrigerated pie … use a clothes dryer as a hiding place … sell both your kidneys on the internet … eat a tube of superglue …' (Dumb Ways to Die 2018b). The final verse made the point that the dumbest ways to die were linked to a lack of safety awareness around trains:

> stand on the edge of a train station platform
> drive around the boom gates at a level crossing
> run across the tracks between the platforms
> they may not rhyme, but they are quite possibly
> the dumbest ways to die …
> *(Tangerine Kitty; cited in Dumb Ways to Die 2018b)*

Designed to promote viral sharability, the video has been viewed over 200 million times on YouTube and the song has sold over 100,000 copies (Dumb Ways to Die 2018a). The campaign was backed-up with posters and images which could be shared on social media, and a set of plush toys available for purchase (Jardine 2017). Two games apps have been developed, the first reaching the number one spot in 22 countries, with over 130 million downloads, and the second follow-up app reaching number one in 83 countries, with 75 million downloads (Dumb Ways to Die 2018a). Most importantly, the campaign seems to have been effective: Metro Trains have recorded a 21 per cent reduction in accidents and deaths on its networks since the campaign started (ibid.).

## Conclusion

Digital public health may appear to be about being 'digital savvy' but the fundamental component of digital public health is still centered around people and around society's efforts to protect and promote the health of communities in the most inclusive and accessible manner. Technology may enable us to do things differently, more efficiently and more effectively, and in a timely manner but, as many of the above examples have shown, digital public health is still about making connections and relationships. Challenging the ingrained and habitual behavior often associated with poor lifestyle choices, requires knowledge and understanding of human motivation. Play is an innate human characteristic and the use of games and ludic creativity to entertain, as well as to give a nudge towards healthier behaviors, is a more positive means of engagement particularly when it also involves opportunities to engage with other people. As a means of skill development and training, games allow us to problem-solve, to try out new strategies, and to make mistakes in a safe environment– all of which promote deep learning that can subsequently be applied in practice. Games are also fun and self-reinforcing and, in this new era of digital public health, it is reassuring to know that 'humans will always want to play, and there's something oddly moving about the lengths to which we will go to invent new games for each other. How touching that, after all this time, we still so badly want to play together' (Hinsliff 2016).

## References

Augment (2018) How Augmented Reality Works, retrieved from www.augment.com/how-augmented-reality-works (accessed 4 March 2018).

Baranowski, T. (2016) Pokémon Go, Go, Go, Gone? *Games for Health Journal*, 5(5): 293–294.

Bartlett, J. (2018) Will 2018 Be the Year of the Neo-luddite? *The Guardian*, 4 March, retrieved from www.theguardian.com/technology/2018/mar/04/will-2018-be-the-year-of-the-neo-luddite (accessed 6 September 2018).

Black, M. (2016) The A–Z of Digital Public Health, retrieved from https://publichealthmatters.blog.gov.uk/2016/07/22/%EF%BB%BFthe-a-z-of-digital-public-health (accessed 6 January 2019).

Black, M. and Dixon, S. (2017) Digital Public Health: 1 February 2017, retrieved from www.wessexphnetwork.org.uk/media/36896/cpd20170201digital-public-health.pdf (accessed 22 February 2018).

Buck, D. and Wenzel, L. (2018) Communities and Health, retrieved from www.kingsfund.org.uk/publications/communities-and-health (accessed 4 March 2018).

Chapman, S. (2017) Pineapples and Stethoscopes: The Problem with Stock Images, retrieved from www.evidentlycochrane.net/stock-images-health-evidence (accessed 26 February 2018).

Digital Unite (2018) How to Plan Intergenerational Activities, retrieved from www.digitalunite.com/spring-online/event-holder-resources/how-plan-intergenerational-activities (accessed 2 March 2018).

Discord (n.d.) Discord Community Guidelines, retrieved from https://discordapp.com/guidelines (accessed 2 September 2018).

Dumb Ways to Die (2018a) Dumb Ways to Die PSA, retrieved from www.dumbwaystodie.com/psa (accessed 3 March 2018).

Dumb Ways to Die (2018b) Dumb Ways to Die – Official Karaoke Version, retrieved from www.dumbwaystodie.com/watch/#video-player (accessed 3 March 2018).

Fitbit League (2017) Hi all Fitbiters, We Are Back Now. Let's Run and Sync with Us, retrieved from www.facebook.com/fitbitleague/posts/2011660005748883 (accessed 2 March 2018).

Fleming, T., Bavin, L., Stasiak, K., Hermansson-Webb, E., Merry, S., Cheek, C., Lucassen, M., Lau, H., Pollmuller, B. and Hetrick, S. (2017) Serious Games and Gamification for Mental Health: Current Status and Promising Directions, *Frontiers in Psychiatry*, retrieved from www.frontiersin.org/articles/10.3389/fpsyt.2016.00215/full (accessed 2 March 2018).

Hinsliff, G. (2016) Why Pokémon Go Really is a National Health Service, *The Guardian*, 22 July, retrieved from www.theguardian.com/commentisfree/2016/jul/22/pokemon-go-health-service-silly-mobile-phone-game-parenting-holy-grail (accessed 23 February 2018).

International Journal of Public Health (2011) Public Health Fun! The Use of Games in Public Health Education, *International Journal of Public Health*, retrieved from http://blogs.springer.com/ijph/food-for-thought/public-health-fun-the-use-of-games-in-public-health-education (accessed 2 March 2018).

Jardine, A. (2017) AdAge 21st Century Ad Campaigns: Metro Trains: Dumb Ways to Die, retrieved from http://adage.com/lp/top15/#dumbways (accessed 23 February 2018).

Johnson, D., Deterdingb, S., Kuhna, K., Stanevaa, A., Stoyanova, S. and Hides, L. (2016) Gamification for Health and Wellbeing: A Systematic Review of the Literature, *Internet Interventions*, 6: 89–106.

Knight, K. (2016) Gamification of Physical Activity: Beat the Street and Pokémon Go, retrieved from www.nesta.org.uk/blog/gamification-physical-activity-beat-street-and-pokemon-go (accessed 23 February 2018).

Malhotra, V. (2012) Role of Game Theory in Public Health, *Journal of Health and Allied Sciences*, 11(2): 2, retrieved from http://cogprints.org/8889/1/2012-2-1.pdf (accessed 1 March 2018).

National Elf Service (2018) About the National Elf Service, retrieved from www.nationalelfservice.net/about-general (accessed 26 February 2018).

Open Forum Events (2018) Digital Transformation: Delivering the Vision for Agile, Flexible and Secure Public Services, retrieved from https://openforumevents.co.uk/events/2018/digital-transformation-delivering-the-vision-for-agile-flexible-and-secure-public-services/#pro (accessed 4 March 2018).

Oxford English Dictionary (2018a) Technology, retrieved from https://en.oxforddictionaries.com/definition/technology (accessed 2 March 2018).

Oxford English Dictionary (2018b) Digital, retrieved from https://en.oxforddictionaries.com/definition/digital (accessed 2 March 2018).

Pappas, C. (2017) Gamification and Serious Games: Differences And Benefits eLearning Pros Need To Know, retrieved from https://elearningindustry.com/gamification-serious-games-differences-benefits-elearning-pros-need-know (accessed 2 March 2018).

Perry, B., Hogan, l. and Marlin, S. (2000) Curiosity, Pleasure and Play: A Neurodevelopmental Perspective, *HAAEYE Advocate*, August: 9–12.

Pflug, K. and Jara, J. (2014) Workplace Fun and Games Motivate Employees, *Workspan*, December: 50–54.

Pokémon Company International (2018) Parents' Guide to Pokémon, retrieved from www.pokemon.com/us/parents-guide (accessed 4 March 2018).

Pravanta, C., Nelson, D. and Harner, R. (2018) *Public Health Communication: Critical Tools and Strategies*, Burlington, VT: Jones & Barlett Learning.

Public Health England (2017) Digital-First Public Health: Public Health England's Digital Strategy, retrieved from www.gov.uk/government/publications/digital-first-public-health/digital-first-public-health-public-health-englands-digital-strategy (accessed 23 February 2018).

RoSPA (2013) *Delivering Accident Prevention at Local Level in the New Public Health System*, Birmingham: Royal Society for the Prevention of Accidents.

RoSPA (2018) Public Health, retrieved from www.rospa.com/public-health (accessed 3 March 2018).

Sailer, M., Ulrich Hense, J., Maya, S. and Mandl, H. (2017) How Gamification Motivates: An Experimental Study of the Effects of Specific Game Design Elements on Psychological Need Satisfaction, *Computers in Human Behavior*, 69: 371–380.

St Ive, I. (2016) *The Unofficial Pokémon GO Field Guide*, London: Weldon Owen.

Schüller, K., Stanková, K. and Thuijsman, F. (2017) Game Theory of Pollution: National Policies and Their International Effects, *Games*, 8: 30, retrieved from www.mdpi.com/2073-4336/8/3/30 (accessed 2 March 2018).

Tomlin, A. and Badenoch, D. (2015) Coping with the Avalanche of Evidence-Based Mental Health Research, retrieved from www.nationalelfservice.net/publication-types/website/coping-with-the-avalanche-of-evidence-based-mental-health-research (accessed 26 February 2018).

UK Government (2016) The UK: Your Partner for Digital Health Solutions, retrieved from www.gov.uk/government/publications/digital-health-working-in-partnership (accessed 26 February 2018).

United Nations (2018) UN E-Government Survey 2016, retrieved from https://publicadm inistration.un.org/egovkb/en-us/Reports/UN-E-Government-Survey-2016 (accessed 23 February 2018).

Van Gool, L. (2016) Ready to Play? The Role of Gamification in Medtech Innovation and Public Health, retrieved from https://medtechengine.com/article/games-for-health (accessed 3 March 2018).

Warner, A. (2016) The Aim of the Game: How the Gamification of Medtech is Putting the Fun into Healthier behaviour, retrieved from https://medtechengine.com/article/gam ification-in-healthcare (accessed 3 March 2018).

Washington, M. (2012) IDIA 620: Information Culture – Dopamine, retrieved from www. slideshare.net/meldawashington/melda-washington-dopamine (accessed 6 March 2018).

Watanabe, K., Kawakami, N., Imamura, K., Inoue, A., Shimazu, A., Yoshikawa, T., Hiro, H., Asai, Y., Odagiri, Y., Yoshikawa, E. and Tsutsumi, A. (2017) Pokémon GO and Psychological Distress, Physical Complaints, and Work Performance among Adult Workers: A Retrospective Cohort Study, *Nature Scientific Reports*, 7: 10758.

Whitaker, J. and Tonkin, A. (2016) Lifespan Development, in A. Tonkin, and J. Whitaker (eds), *Play in Healthcare for Adults: Using Play to Promote Health and Wellbeing Across the Adult Lifespan*, 32–44, Abingdon: Routledge.

Winslow, C. (1920) The Untilled Fields of Public Health, *Science*, 51(1306): 23–33.

World Health Organization (2016) *Monitoring and Evaluating Digital Health Interventions: A Practical Guide to Conducting Research and Assessment*, Geneva: World Health Organization.

World Health Organization (2018) The Public Health Approach, retrieved from www.who. int/violenceprevention/approach/public_health/en (accessed 22 February 2018).

Yuen, S. (2018) I Think @PokemonGoApp is an Awesome Example … Twitter, 6 March, retrieved from https://twitter.com/S3bster/status/970921282278653952?s=19 (accessed 6 September 2018).

Zeroghan (2018) Norwegian Prime Minister 'Caught' Playing Pokémon GO Before a Meeting with Trump, retrieved from https://pokemongohub.net/post/news/norwegia n-prime-minister-caught-playing-pokemon-go-meeting-trump (accessed 4 March 2018).

# 12

# A PLACE FOR PLAY

## Creating playful environments for health and wellbeing

*Julia Whitaker and Alison Tonkin*

## Introduction

In 2017, Bird et al. were commissioned by Public Health England to explore the impact on health of natural and built environments, by collating evidence from a variety of perspectives to illustrate the associations 'between planning principles, health impact and health-related outcomes' (Bird et al. 2017). Natural and built environments cover the broad spectrum of physical environments in which 'people live, work and play, including: schools, workplaces, homes, communities, and parks/ recreation areas, green spaces (i.e. visible grass, trees and other vegetation) and blue spaces (i.e. visible water)' (ibid.: 7). The report clearly identified the significance of both the natural and built environment as key determinants of health and wellbeing, while acknowledging the subjective and individualistic nature of how environments are experienced by individuals, communities and society as a whole (ibid.).

The impact of environmental considerations on children's play is well established (International Play Association 2016) and there is a growing recognition that for children (and adults) to reap the benefits of play, the environments in which we live need to be conducive to playful activity. The International Play Association (ibid.) defines play as a process which is non-compulsory, intrinsically motivated and undertaken for pleasure, with no defined outcome. The play environment should provide challenge, be flexible and adaptive and, most importantly, fun. In this context, play facilitates the development of autonomy and promotes physical, mental and emotional activity at both individual and group levels (ibid.). The International Play Association (ibid.: 2) sees play as a 'particular way of engaging with the world' and states that 'while playing, children [and adults] can experience the vitality of a range of emotions, with less consequence than such emotions may bring in the "real" world. This can give rise to positive feelings and pleasure, a sense that life is worth living for the time of playing.'

This chapter will explore the relationship between play, health and the environment, using the concepts of *playful setting* and *playscape to* contrast natural and built environments. It will discuss the role of the environment in shaping opportunities for play and playfulness, while acknowledging that sometimes it is just time and space that are needed for play to flow freely. It will also discuss how enhanced environments can impact on people's behaviors, attitudes and perceptions (Bird et al. 2017), particularly when they incorporate elements of play and playfulness. The chapter reflects recognition of the impact of how and where we live on the public health agenda.

## Contextualizing the playful environment

An environmental approach to public health is embodied in the Ottawa Charter for Health Promotion (World Health Organization 1986) which advocated community participation, partnership, empowerment and equity for the creation of the *'healthy settings'* which would lead to the improvement of public health worldwide. The World Health Organization defines a setting for health as: 'the place or social context in which people engage in daily activities in which environmental, organizational, and personal factors interact to affect health and wellbeing' (World Health Organization 1998).

A settings-based approach to health long pre-dates the Ottawa Charter. The work of the Greek physician Hippocrates (460–370 BCE), *'Airs, Waters, and Places'*, is thought to be the first systematic attempt to set-out the relationship between human health and the environment. Hippocrates recognized that certain physical and mental characteristics were reflective of where people lived, worked and played. Historical attempts to create 'healthy settings' have typically been community initiatives following a pattern which has become familiar in modern public health provision: creative initiative generates public opinion which attracts governmental attention and cues demand for governmental action. A 'settings' approach thus emphasizes the individual, social and systemic dimensions of health promotion (Poland et al. 2000) and a 'whole systems' model recognizes the confluence of history, culture and social structure in the biography of place as it relates to public health (Poland and Dooris 2010).

The Healthy Cities movement is probably the most widely recognized example of the healthy settings approach. A *healthy city* is defined as 'one that continually creates and improves its physical and social environments and expands the community resources that enable people to mutually support each other in performing all the functions of life and developing to their maximum potential' (World Health Organization 2018). A key feature of the Healthy Cities movement is that it does not prescribe or advocate specific policies but emphasizes process and local context over particular activities (Werna et al. 1999) allowing for a broad interpretation of 'healthy'. Hancock and Duhl (1988) state that any city can be a healthy city since this is not a status definition but the description of a process, the purpose of which is to improve population health and health equity. Thirty years after the launch of the Healthy Cities movement in 1986, thousands of cities are part of the Healthy Cities network and exist in all World Health Organization regions and in more than 1,000 countries worldwide.

The original model of the healthy setting, associated with the Ottawa charter and the healthy cities movement, has been 'revitalized' with the advance of the 'supersetting approach' (Bloch et al. 2014) which argues that health promotion activities may be optimized through the integrated efforts of public, private and voluntary sectors and civic society. Based on ecological and whole-systems thinking, the idea of the 'supersetting' embodies and extends the principles of participation, empowerment, context and knowledge-based development necessary for the nurturance of a culture of health. A dynamic example of a supersetting is the 'playful setting', which represents the realization of people power in the creative pursuit of healthful change.

## Playful settings

The global adoption of the healthy settings approach, and the widespread acceptance of the significance of green space, has been matched by the growth of a worldwide movement for play, and the notion of the 'playful setting' as conducive to health and wellbeing. There appear to be dual motivations for the creation of playful settings, which can be explained in terms of the 'arts and health diamond' of McNaughton et al. (2005). This model recognizes the overlap between the intended and unintended consequences of any societal intervention for individual or community wellbeing. Firstly, there is the direct motivation that play, particularly physical play, can make a valuable contribution to public health efforts to reduce the global health burdens of inactivity and obesity. A playful setting correlates to a healthy setting when it permits, promotes and supports physical activity. There is also the indirect motivation that play and playfulness are valued as mediators of social interaction, social harmony and subjective wellbeing, with positive implications for both personal and public health. When we play, we 'feel' better and the feeling of subjective wellbeing acts as a driver for healthful action (Impact Arts 2011).

## The 'playscape'

Frost (1992) coined the term 'playscape' to describe an environment which is specifically designed, or designated, as a place to play. While the term has become associated with contemporary play spaces which integrate design elements with the natural surroundings, the idea of a separate but integral space for play originated at the end of the 19th century with German 'sand gardens' (O'Shea, 2013). However, the traditional 'playscape' has always been the street or village where people lived-out their day-to-day lives. Historically, the street was not only a living playground for neighborhood children, but also a social center, where adults of all ages could socialize in close proximity to their homes and children (Cowman 2017). However, over the course of the second half of the twentieth century, the street as playscape has been largely usurped by commercial enterprise and motor traffic. Long working hours, increased educational demands, and the expansion of professional childcare, as well as safety concerns, have gradually restricted the use of the street as a shared space for play and social interaction, to the detriment of public health and wellbeing (Page et al. 2017).

'Playing out' in the street and in the surrounding neighborhood creates opportunities for people of different generations and cultures to mix in a safe and positive way, with all the associated benefits for physical, psychological and social health (see www.aplayfulcity.com). The United Nations (2013) recognizes that the shared experience of inclusive public spaces by different age groups serves to promote and strengthen civil society while encouraging children to recognize themselves as citizens with rights – including the right to be healthy (Article 24) and the right to play (Article 31). The United Nations (2013) advocates children's play as ' fundamental to the quality of childhood, to children's entitlement to optimum development, to the promotion of resilience, and to the realization of other rights' (ibid.: III.8). It is the responsibility of national and local government to 'respect, fulfil and protect' (ibid.) the right to play and recreation for all children and young people, and Voce (2018) argues that this means 'they should adopt measures to legislate, budget and plan for children's play'.

Reclaiming the street as a playscape is being promoted around the world by grassroots organizations such as 'Playing Out' (http://playingout.net) in Bristol in the UK and 'Te Veo en la Calle' (http://te-veo.org) in Bilbao, Spain. The 'Open Streets' project (http://openstreetsproject.org) in the US and initiatives such as 'A Playful Street' (www.aplayfulcity.com/the-lab) in Dublin, Ireland extend the idea of street play as a cultural resource for all members of the community.

Landscape architects and designers have adopted playscape terminology to define the environmental features that encourage play and social interaction for all age-groups (Fjørtoft and Sageie 2000). Key to the concept of the playscape is that it is a space perceived by the players as offering possibilities for play. Boon et al. (2015) have elucidated four essential qualities of a playscape:

- It recognizes the spatial qualities of play, taking the play beyond dedicated boundaries.
- It is a landscape to *move through,* rather than a destination, and as such prompts physical play.
- It is a locus for open-ended activity, allowing for a diverse interpretation of what constitutes play and playfulness and leading to a sense of ownership of the play within the space.
- It offers a sense of '*placeness*' – 'a degree of containment that serves to separate off the rest of the world' (Talbot and Frost 1990: 229) – which encourages attachment to place and sustained engagement in the play.

Exploring and playing in a playscape involves physical movement: the use of gross motor and perceptual skills such as spatial and directional awareness. An experimental study by Fjørtoft (2004) found that the benefits to physical fitness, balance and coordination were enhanced when the playscape was a natural environment rather than a more traditional play setting. Opportunities for social interaction within the playscape also nurture social and emotional development (Fjørtoft and Sageie 2000). Having a 'sense of place' for play is reflected in the development of self-identity, traditions, connections and memories (Jivén and Larkham 2003) and in a sense of personal investment in the natural environment. The Roman poet, Ovid (427–347 BCE) wrote, 'In our play we reveal what kind of people we are' (Goodreads 2018): the incorporation of playscapes within the healthy settings approach offers not only potential benefits for both physical health and for social and emotional wellbeing, but for the process of transition towards a sustainable culture of health.

## Going green – exploring the natural environment

Physical inactivity is the fourth largest cause of disease and death in the UK (Parliamentary Office of Science and Technology 2016). It has been estimated that one in four women and one in five men spend less than the recommended 30 minutes per day engaged in physical activity (Benwell et al. 2013), and one in four children spend less than 30 minutes playing outside per week (Moss 2012).

Levels of physical activity have been directly linked to access to 'green space': natural or semi-natural areas occurring in or near urban areas, including parks, woodlands and allotments, which provide habitat for wildlife and can be used for recreation. Physical activity levels are highest in areas with more green space, and people living near the greenest areas are most likely to achieve recommended activity levels (Mytton et al. 2012). In green space, natural materials can blend with the exercise regime. For example, in 2016, the National Trust commissioned an outdoor gym, shown in Figure 12.1, which integrates 'their principles of conservation and sustainability into [our] design, keeping visual disruption to the landscape to a minimum and impacting as little as possible on the local natural environment' (Boex 2016). The use of the natural environment for promoting exercise has been fully embraced by the Parkrun movement, which organizes free, timed, 5km weekly runs for anyone who wants to participate (see www.parkrun. org.uk). There are currently over 556 locations in the UK where these runs take place in 'pleasant parkland surroundings'. Since the first Parkrun at the end of 2005, which had 109 'athletes', there are now more than 130,000 people regularly doing these runs, facilitated by over 11,000 volunteers (Parkrun UK 2018).

Studies in the Netherlands have linked better access to green space to increased perceived health and to the reduced prevalence of diseases such as diabetes (Maas et al. 2009). In the UK, a correlation has been observed between those living closest to greener areas and reduced levels of mortality, obesity and obesity-related illnesses (Hillsdon et al. 2011). Notably, health inequalities are halved in greener areas: a 2010 study suggests that among those at greatest socio-economic disadvantage, mortality rates are halved in areas with the greenest space (Marmot 2010). Mitchell et al. (2015) also found that socioeconomic inequality in mental wellbeing was 40 per cent narrower among people reporting good access to green or recreational areas, compared to those with poor access.

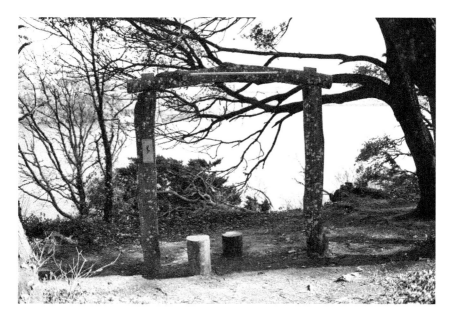

**FIGURE 12.1** National Trust green outdoor gym at Loe Pool.
Source: Boex (2016); photograph by Will Boex

It is evident from the research that the benefits of interacting with green space extend beyond the physical domain, to the social and emotional aspects of health. It has been shown that physical activity in a natural setting reduces blood pressure and raises subjective wellbeing compared with a similar level of activity in an urban environment (Bird 2007). Control trials have also found that people exercising outdoors report higher feelings of wellbeing, and lower feelings of stress or anxiety, than those doing the same activity indoors (Thompson Coon et al. 2011). There is further evidence that engagement with nature has a positive impact on mental health, improving cognitive function and reducing anxiety for those living with conditions such as ADHD, depression and dementia (Bragg and Atkins 2016). Improvements in mood, self-esteem and physical fitness have also been reported by ecotherapy projects (Mind 2013), which incorporate the combined benefits of nature, physical activity, mental wellbeing, social interaction, and inclusion (Jordan and Hinds 2016).

The natural environment offers many possibilities for play and, as such, represents a 'natural playscape'. Play in nature invites curiosity and awakens the imagination and a sense of wonder, nurturing connectedness and affinity with the local ecology (Izenstark and Ebata 2014), with benefits for social and emotional wellness. Compared with other recreational activities, play in nature is perceived as more fun, relaxing, and interesting and has been shown to contribute to improved filial interaction (Izenstark and Ebata 2017).

The Japanese art of *shinrin-yoku* or 'forest-bathing' – spending time in nature, among trees – has been shown to have a positive impact on physical and mental health, even in the absence of intentional physical exercise. Scientific studies by Li (2018) have shown that forest-bathing improves the immune system; increases energy levels; reduces stress, depression and anxiety; and promotes overall feelings of relaxation and wellbeing. These findings have resulted in the creation of 62 certified forest-therapy bases in Japan, and between 2.5 and 5 million people have been encouraged to walk the forest trails every year (Li 2018). Other parts of the world are now also beginning to value the potential of forest bathing, 'with its power to touch all five senses and provide a natural boost to well-being' (D'Silva 2018: 64).

## Green city: healthy city

A green city is a healthy city: accessible and attractive green space can provide safe and pleasurable opportunities for urban residents to enjoy physical activity and recreation, to engage in social interaction, and to relieve the stresses of daily life. The evidence demonstrates that green space offers particular benefits to economically disadvantaged communities (Mitchell et al. 2015), to children (Richardson et al. 2017), to pregnant women (Grazuleviciene et al. 2015), and to the elderly (e.g. Marshall and Gilliard 2014; Cherrie et al. 2018). Cities with green space are likely to have healthier citizens and therefore reduced demands on health services, contributing to a robust economy.

The global initiative 'Healthy Parks, Healthy People' acknowledges that contact with nature is essential for human emotional, physical and spiritual health and well-being, and reinforces the crucial role played by parks and protected green space in nurturing healthy ecosystems (Healthy Parks Healthy People 2015). Healthy Parks, Healthy People recognizes a global responsibility for creating opportunities for children and young people to experience and connect with nature in ways that are meaningful for them. A study by Veitch et al. (2016) explored this 'meaningfulness' in terms of the features of parks which make them most appealing to adolescents, and these over-whelmingly represented opportunities for play. A further experimental study of the impact of the installation of a designed playscape, demonstrated its potential to increase park visitation and park-based physical activity (Veitch et al. 2018).

The 'Park Prescriptions' movement (Seltenrich 2015) is a US initiative which integrates park visits into medical treatment and prevention plans. There appear to be two avenues through which green space is likely promote improved physical and mental health. The first is nature's mentally restorative quality, evidenced by the research into Japanese forest-bathing (Li 2018). The second is the social cohesion achieved through spending time outdoors with family, friends, and fellow citizens (Triguero-Mas et al. 2015). Green space shares these qualities with play which also restores mental balance (Scarlett et al. 2005) and promotes social closeness (Youell 2008). Where the qualities of play and of green space coalesce in the natural playscape, the holistic benefits to health are multiplied (e.g. Bento and Dias 2017).

Parks are public spaces and all members of the community should have equal and equitable access to green space with its associated health benefits. The subject of urban green space is embedded in the European health policy framework, Health 2020 (World Health Organization 2013), in the context of creating resilient communities and supportive environments. The Parma Declaration (World Health Organization 2010) commits by 2020 'to provide each child with access … to green spaces in which to play and undertake physical activity'. The 2030 Agenda for Sustainable Development (United Nations 2015), which pledges to 'leave no one behind', set the following goal: 'by 2030 to provide universal access to safe, inclusive and accessible, green and public spaces, in particular for women and children, older persons and persons with disabilities'.

## Exploring the built environment

Human behavior is heavily context dependent and even small changes to our surroundings can influence how we feel (Dolan et al. 2016). The built environment – 'places and spaces created or modified by people including buildings, parks, and transportation systems' (Health Canada 2002) – has a significant influence on behavior, much of which is unconscious. In recognition of this, all new built environments would ideally factor into their design specific features which impact on wellbeing. Dolan et al. (2016) have developed a checklist for design using the mnemonic SALIENT – sound, air, light, image, ergonomics, nature and tint – and identify numerous examples of how each of these elements can be used to influence our behavior – both consciously and unconsciously, as shown in Table 12.1.

When designing built environments, the SALIENT checklist provides a useful tool for ensuring that consideration of health and wellbeing are integrated into the planning process.

## The playful city

Play and playfulness can be 'built into' the design of new environments to a similar end. The concept of the 'Playable City' expands the idea of playscape by putting play at the heart of future city design, 're-using city infrastructure and re-appropriating smart city technologies to create connections – person to person, person to city' (see www.playablecity.com). Launched in Bristol in the UK in 2012, Playable City is active internationally in cities as diverse as Tokyo, Recife and Austin, Texas. Reflecting the manifold nature of play, each playable city network engages in a culturally-specific way with the issues and opportunities present in their own locale.

A recent example of a Playable City project is the 'Stop Smile Stroll' installation in Bristol, which transforms pedestrian crossings into opportunities for playful social interaction, connecting strangers for 30 seconds of shared fun in the course of the daily commute (Arts Council England 2016). Another playful project, 'Playful Welcome' in Japan, is an international collaboration developing playful ideas to connect visitors and local people to each other during the Olympic and Paralympic

**TABLE 12.1** SALIENT key insights.

| Element | Effect | Considerations |
|---|---|---|
| Sound | Our attention is drawn to unpredictable and attention seeking sounds. | Music is known to have significant influence on our moods and can be used to facilitate calmness or enhance concentration. |
| Air | We are affected by air flow, temperature, source and scents. | Good ventilation, freedom from air pollution, and the use of scent can boost our sense of wellness. |
| Light | Our behavior is influenced by the source and brightness of light. | Natural light is preferable to artificial light, while dim light enhances creativity. Imagery, in the form of visual art or prints, actively promotes health and wellbeing. |
| Image | We are stimulated by certain imagery and affected by clutter | Cluttered surroundings can lead to distraction, which is particularly difficult for people with dementia. |
| Ergonomics | We do not adapt well to poorly designed furniture and equipment | Poorly designed furniture and equipment is known to be detrimental to health and wellbeing, while the use of uncomfortable safety equipment means it is less likely to be used. |
| Nature | We are affected in largely positive ways by exposure to natural elements. | The incorporation of nature into the built environment has significant links to wellbeing: the use of indoor plants increases attention span, while images of nature and natural elements such as air, light and sound have a positive impact on health and wellbeing. |
| Tint | Our behavior is affected by the presence of different colors. | Tint, or the use of color, affects behavior largely at an unconscious level and the therapeutic use of color has long been associated with healing, health and wellbeing, dating back to the ancient civilizations (Color Therapy n.d.). |

Source: adapted from Dolan et al. (2016: 2)

Games in 2020. The Playable City concept can also be applied to issues of serious global concern, such as air pollution. In 2018, artist Michael Pinsky installed five geodesic domes in the forecourt of Somerset House in London, each one containing a different simulated atmospheric environment. Visitors moved through the pods, experiencing the contrast between the fresh, clean air of Tautra in Norway and the highly polluted atmospheres of London, New Delhi, Beijing and Sao Paolo. Pinsky's work invites visitors to consider the complex and interconnected nature of the global community, using a playful approach to challenge perceptions of climate change in a more meaningful way than conventional media (Power 2018).

Despite the cultural disparities created by the local context of Playable City projects, they are united by three key principles (Baggini 2014). Firstly, they concede that the problems associated with urban living can only be addressed by collective action. Secondly, they acknowledge that change is the shared responsibility of the individual and the state. Thirdly, Playable City represents an optimism that playful public activities can contribute to a happier, more cohesive, urban future (ibid.). Public health rests on the premise of social justice (Kreiger and Birn 1998) and it is the universal desire to 'make the world a better place' for all that continues to prompt innovative endeavor. Play and playfulness interrupt the functional efficiency of the modern urban environment, reminding us of our shared humanity (Baggini 2014).

The pertinence of the playful setting for public health rests on two principles embedded in play theory: *permission* and *choice*. Firstly, people (whether children or adults) need to feel that they have permission to engage in the play and that they will not be judged negatively for doing so (De Koven 2016). Huizinga (1955) used the image of the 'magic circle' to describe a place for play which is both in the real world and separate from it (physically or metaphorically) – a 'safe' place to play where conventional codes of conduct do not apply and where new behaviors, beliefs, and interactions become not only possible but permissible (Whitton 2018). However, Whitton (2018) cautions that the creation of safe places for play demands more than simply permission or invitation to play: playful settings need to be shaped over a period of time, during which players build the trust and develop the relationships which make play possible.

The second principle underlying the 'playful healthy setting' is that of *choice*. Play is always voluntary and intrinsically motivated, otherwise it becomes something other than 'playful'. Participation in play is motivated by the internal reward system (Perry et al. 2000), rather than by any external incentive or enticement. Whitton (2018) explains: 'intrinsically motivated engagement creates the capacity for personal exploration, experimentation and discovery, leading to learning that is personally meaningful.' Play is largely defined by the choice and control that people enjoy while playing: if players are not free to choose what to do or how to do it, then an activity may be *play-full* but it cannot truly be called *play* (Voce 2018)

Volkswagen's 'fun theory' of behavior change tests this idea, based on the assumption that playful physical activity can serve to benefit public health if it is perceived as 'fun', and is freely chosen by the participants. 'Piano Stairs' was an interactive musical stairway installed alongside the escalator at the Odenplan subway station in Stockholm to encourage passengers to use the stairs more often. Studies show that, when offered the choice between climbing stairs or taking the escalator, commuters choose to take the stairs 66 percent more often if they are piano stairs (Rolighetsteorin 2009). The Piano Stairs concept has now been replicated around the world from Milan to Shanghai, using playfulness to achieve a healthful change in behavior. The piano metaphor for play reappears in Edinburgh in 2018 with the installation of the world's first *pianodrome* – a 100-seater amphitheatre constructed entirely from upcycled pianos as 'a place for all to play' in more than one sense of

the word: five of the pianos are tuned for visitors to play music (see www.pia
nodrome.co.uk)!

Creative initiatives are to be celebrated but for the playable city to thrive it
requires cooperation from local government. Baggini (2014) writes:

> There are very clear incentives for councils to come on board. Since Rome,
> legislators have acknowledged that a thriving metropolis requires bread and
> circuses, more than just the bare essentials. Many of the playable city ideas
> provide very cheap ways of doing this.

Marmot (2010) affirms that physical and social landscapes, and the degree to which
they prompt and facilitate healthy behaviors, are key to creating an equitable culture of health.

## Conclusion

The spontaneity of play means it can and does happen anywhere and at any time. The
natural environment enhances wellbeing by its very presence, offering space and a
sense of being at one with nature. Natural settings can also be adapted to facilitate
physical activity and playful endeavors, both of which contribute to physical and
mental health. Games played in informal settings demonstrate the flexibility of play,
altering in response to the materials available, the skills of the players and their play
preferences – all of which are influenced by the environment in which the play takes
place (De Koven 2016). From localized street play to the design of playful cities, play
transforms the built environment, enriching all our lives. Play and health share a
symbiotic relationship and public health measures must recognize that an environment
which incorporates 'a place to play' is more likely to become a healthy place to live.

## References

Arts Council England (2016) Transforming Pedestrian Crossings into Playful Moments,
   retrieved    from    www.artscouncil.org.uk/news/transforming-pedestrian-crossings-pla
   yful-moments (accessed 21 July 2018).
Baggini, J. (2014) Playable Cities: The City That Plays Together, Stays Together, retrieved
   from    www.theguardian.com/cities/2014/sep/04/playable-cities-the-city-that-plays-to
   gether-stays-together (accessed 21 July 2018).
Bento, G. and Dias, G. (2017) The Importance of Outdoor Play for Young Children's
   Healthy Development, Porto Biomedical Journal, 2(5): 157–160.
Benwell, R., Burfield, P., Hardiman, A., McCarthy, D., Marsh, S., Middleton, J., Morling,
   P., Wilkinson, P. and Wynde, R. (2013) A Nature and Wellbeing Act, Sandy: RSPB.
Bird, W., 2007, Natural Thinking: Investigating the Links Between the Natural Environment,
   Biodiversity and Mental Health, Sandy: RSPB.
Bird, E., Ige, J., Burgess-Allen, J., Pinto, A. and Pilkington, P. (2017) Spatial Planning for
   Health: An Evidence Resource for Planning and Designing Healthier Places: Full Technical Report,
   Bristol: University of the West of England.

Bloch, P., Toft, U., Reinbach, H. C., Clausen, L. T., Mikkelsen, B. E., Poulsen, K. and Jensen, B. (2014) Revitalizing the Setting Approach – Supersettings for Sustainable Impact in Community Health Promotion. *The International Journal of Behavioral Nutrition and Physical Activity*, 11: 118.

Boex (2016) National Trust Outdoor Gym, retrieved from www.boex.co.uk/portfolio/national-trust-outdoor-gym (accessed 24 August 2018).

Boon, B., Rozendaal, M. and Stappers, P. (2015) Playscapes as a Design Perspective on Children's Physical Play and Wellbeing, retrieved from www.researchgate.net/publication/274696067_Playscapes_as_a_Design_Perspective_on_Children%27s_Physical_Play_and_Wellbeing (accessed 17 July 2018).

Bragg, R. and Atkins, G. (2016) *A Review of Nature-Based Interventions for Mental Health Care*, York: Natural England.

Cherrie, M., Shortt, N., Mitchell, R., Taylor, A., Redmond, P., Ward Thompson, C., Starr, J., Deary, I. and Pearce, J. (2018) Green Space and Cognitive Ageing: A Retrospective Life Course Analysis in the Lothian Birth Cohort 1936. *Social Science and Medicine*, 196: 56–65.

Colour Therapy (n.d) What is Colour Therapy?, retrieved from www.colourtherapyhealing.com/colour-therapy/what-colour-therapy (accessed 24 August 2018).

Cowman, K. (2017) Play Streets: Women, Children and the Problem of Urban Traffic, 1930–1970. *Social History*, 42(2): 233–256.

De Koven, B. L. (2016) The Playful Life, retrieved from www.aplayfulpath.com/playful-life (accessed 23 July 2018).

Dolan, P., Foy, C. and Smith, S. (2016) The SALIENT Checklist: Gathering up the Ways in Which Built Environments Affect What We Do and How We Feel, *Buildings*, 6(9): 1–8.

D'Silva, B. (2018) A sea of green, *Breathe*, 10: 64–67.

Fjørtoft, I. (2004) Landscape as Playscape: The Effects of Natural Environments on Children's Play and Motor Development, *Children, Youth and Environments*, 14(2): 21–44.

Fjørtoft, I. and Sageie, J. (2000) The Natural Environment as a Playground for Children: Landscape Description and Analyses of a Natural Playscape, *Landscape and Urban Planning*, 48(1–2): 83–97.

Frost, J. L. (1992) *Play and Playscapes*, New York: Delmar.

Goodreads (2018) Ovid Quotes, retrieved from www.goodreads.com/quotes/96824-in-our-play-we-reveal-what-kind-of-people-we (accessed 27 August 2018).

Grazuleviciene, R., Danileviciute, A., Dedele, A., Vencloviene, J., Andrusaityte, S., Uždanaviciute, I., and Nieuwenhuijsen, M. J. (2015) Surrounding Greenness, Proximity to City Parks and Pregnancy Outcomes in Kaunas Cohort Study, *International Journal of Hygiene and Environmental Health*, 218(3), 358–365.

Hancock, T. .and Duhl, I. (1988) *Promoting Health in the Urban Context*, World Health Organization Healthy Cities Papers, no. 1, Copenhagen: FADL.

Health Canada (2002) *Natural and Built Environments*, Ottawa: Health Canada.

Healthy Parks, Healthy People (2015) *A Guide to the Healthy Parks Healthy People Approach and Current Practices: Proceedings from the Improving Health and Well-being: Healthy Parks Healthy People Stream of the IUCN World Parks Congress 2014*, Melbourne: Parks Victoria.

Hillsdon, M., Jones, A. and Coombes, E., 2011, *Green Space Access, Green Space Use, Physical Activity and Overweight*, York: Natural England.

Huizinga, J. (1955) *Homo Ludens: A Study of the Play Element in Culture*, Boston, MA: Beacon Press.

Impact Arts (2011) *Craft Café. Social Return on Investment Evaluation*, Glasgow: Social Value Lab.

International Play Association (2016) Children's Right to Play and the Environment, retrieved from http://ipaworld.org/wp-content/uploads/2016/05/IPA-Play-Environment-Discussion-Paper.pdf (accessed 23 August 2018).

Izenstark, D. and Ebata, A. (2014) Connecting Children and Families to Nature: An Evaluation of a Natural Playscape, *Parks and Recreation Magazine*, 6: 62–66.

Izenstark, D. and Ebata, A. (2017) The Effects of the Natural Environment on Attention and Family Cohesion: An Experimental Study, *Children, Youth and Environments*, 27(2): 93–109.

Jivén, G. and Larkham, P. J. (2003) Sense of Place, Authenticity and Character: A Commentary, *Journal of Urban Design*, 8(1): 67–81.

Jordan, M. and Hinds, J. (eds) (2016) *Ecotherapy: Theory, Research and Practice*, London: Macmillan.

Kreiger, N. and Birn, A. E. (1998) A Vision of Social Justice as the Foundation of Public Health: Commemorating 150 Years of the Spirit of 1848, *American Journal of Public Health*, 88(11): 1603–1606.

Li, Q. (2018) *Forest Bathing: How Trees Can Help You Find Health and Happiness*, New York: Viking.

Maas, J., Verheij, R., de Vries, S., Spreeuwenberg, P., Schellevis, F.G., and Groenewegen, P. (2009) Morbidity is Related to a Green Living Environment, *Journal of Epidemiology and Community Health*, 63(12): 967–973.

McNaughton, J., White, M. and Stacey, R. (2005) Researching the Benefits of Arts in Health, *Health Education*, 105(5): 332–339.

Marmot, M. (2010) *Fair Society Healthy Lives (Full Report)*, London: Marmot Review.

Marshall, M. and Gilliard, J. (eds) (2014) *Creating Culturally Appropriate Outside Spaces and Experiences for People with Dementia: Using Nature and the Outdoors in Person-Centred Care*, London: Jessica Kingsley Publishers.

Mind (2013) *Feel Better Outside, Feel Better Inside: Ecotherapy for Mental Wellbeing, Resilience and Recovery*, London: Mind.

Mitchell, R., Richard, E., Shortt, N. and Pearce, J. (2015) Neighborhood Environments and Socioeconomic Inequalities in Mental Well-Being, *American Journal of Preventive Medicine*, 49(1): 80–84.

Moss, S. (2012) *Natural Childhood*, retrieved from www.nationaltrust.org.uk/documents/read-our-natural-childhood-report.pdf (accessed 18 July 2018).

Mytton, O., Townsend, N., Rutter, H. and Foster, C. (2012) Green Space and Physical Activity: An Observational Study Using Health Survey for England Data, *Health & Place*, 18(5): 1034–1041.

O'Shea, K., (2013) How We Came to Play: The History of Playgrounds, retrieved from https://savingplaces.org/stories/how-we-came-to-play-the-history-of-playgrounds/#.W1lwWvZFzIU (accessed 26 July 2018).

Page, A., Cooper, A., Hampton, L., Read, J. and Tibbitts, B. (2017) *Why Temporary Street Closures for Play Make Sense for Public Health*, London: Play England.

Parkrun UK (2018) Historical Chart of Number of Parkrun Event, Parkrunners and Volunteers, retrieved from www.parkrun.org.uk/results/historicalchart (accessed 24 August 2018).

Parliamentary Office of Science and Technology (2016) Green Space and Health, retrieved from http://researchbriefings.files.parliament.uk/documents/POST-PN-0538/POST-PN-0538.pdf (accessed 18 July 2018).

Perry, B., Hogan, l. and Marlin, S. (2000) Curiosity, Pleasure and Play: A Neurodevelopmental Perspective, *HAAEYE Advocate*, August: 9–12.

Poland, B. and Dooris, M. (2010) A Green and Healthy Future: The Settings Approach to Building Health, Equity, and Sustainability, *Critical Public Health*, 20: 281–298.

Poland, B., Green, L. and Rootman, I. (2000) *Settings for Health Promotion: Linking Theory and Practice*, London: Sage.

Power, S. (2018) Michael Pinsky: Pollution Pods, retrieved from www.somersethouse.org.uk/whats-on/michael-pinsky-pollution-pods (accessed 21 July 2018).

Richardson, E.A., Pearce, J., Short, N.K. and Mitchell, R. (2017) The Role of Public and Private Natural Space in Children's Social, Emotional, and behavioural Development in Scotland: A Longitudinal Study, *Environmental Research*, 158: 729–736.

Rolighetsteorin (2009) Piano Stairs, retrieved from www.youtube.com/watch?v=2lXh2n0a Pyw (accessed 22 July 2018).

Scarlett, W., Naudeau, S., Salonius-Pasternak, D. and Ponte, I. (2005) Restorative Play in Stressful Environments, in W. Scarlett, S. Naudeau, D. Salonius-Pasternak and I. Ponte (eds), *Children's Play*, 201–230, Thousand Oaks, CA: Sage Publications.

Seltenrich, N. (2015) Just What the Doctor Ordered: Using Parks to Improve Children's Health, *Environmental Health Perspectives*, 123(10): 254–259.

Talbot, J. and Frost, J. (1990) Magical Playscapes, in S. Wortham and J. Frost (eds), *Playgrounds for Young Children: National Survey and Perspectives*, 224–243, Reston, VA: American Alliance for Health, Physical Education, Recreation and Dance.

Thompson Coon, J., Boddy, K., Stein, K., Whear, R., Barton, J. and Depledge, M. (2011) Does Participating in Physical Activity in Outdoor Natural Environments Have a Greater Effect on Physical and Mental Wellbeing than Physical Activity Indoors? A Systematic Review, *Environmental Science and Technology*, 45: 1761–1772.

Triguero-Mas, M., Dadvand, P., Cirach, M., Martínez, D., Medina, A., Mompart, A., Basagaña, X., Gražulevičienė, R. and Nieuwenhuijsen, M.J. (2015) Natural Outdoor Environments and Mental and Physical Health: Relationships and Mechanisms, *Environment International*, 77: 35–41.

United Nations (2013) *General Comment No. 17 (2013) on the Right of the Child to Rest, Leisure, Play, Recreational Activities, Cultural Life and the Arts (Art. 31)*, New York: United Nations.

United Nations (2015) Transforming Our World: The 2030 Agenda for Sustainable Development, retrieved from https://sustainabledevelopment.un.org/content/documents/21252030%20Agenda%20for%20Sustainable%20Development%20web.pdf (accessed 19 July 2018).

Veitch, J., Salmon, J., Crawford, D., Abbott, G., Giles-Corti, B., Carver, A. and Timperio, A. (2018) The REVAMP Natural Experiment Study: The Impact of a Play-scape Installation on Park Visitation and Park-Based Physical Activity, *International Journal of Behavioral Nutrition and Physical Activity*, 15: 10.

Veitch, J., Salmon, J., Parker, K., Bangay, S., Deforche, B., and Timperio, A. (2016) Adolescents' Ratings of Features of Parks that Encourage Park Visitation and Physical Activity, *International Journal of Behavioral Nutrition and Physical Activity*, 13: 73.

Voce, A. (2018) What Do We Mean by a Playful City?, retrieved from www.aplayfulcity.com/single-post/2018/01/29/1-Why-should-cities-aim-to-be-playful (accessed 25 July 2018).

Werna, E., Harpham, T., Blue, I. and Goldstein, G. (1998) *Healthy City Projects in Developing Countries: An International Approach to Local Problems*, London: Earthscan.

Whitton, N. (2018) Playful Learning: Tools, Techniques, and Tactics, *Research in Learning Technology*, 26: 2035retrieved from https://journal.alt.ac.uk/index.php/rlt/article/view/2035/html (accessed 27 August 2018).

World Health Organization, (1986) *The Ottawa Charter for Health Promotion*, Geneva: World Health Organization.

World Health Organization (1998) *Health Promotion Glossary*, Geneva: World Health Organization.

World Health Organization (2010) Parma Declaration on Environment and Health, retrieved from www.euro.who.int/__data/assets/pdf_file/0011/78608/E93618.pdf (accessed 19 July 2018).

World Health Organization (2013) *Health 2020: A European Policy Framework Supporting Action across Government and Society for Health and Well-being*, Geneva: World Health Organization.

World Health Organization (2018) What is a Healthy City?, retrieved from www.euro.who.int/en/health-topics/environment-and-health/urban-health/who-european-healthy-cities-network/what-is-a-healthy-city (accessed 24 July 2018).

Youell, B. (2008) The Importance of Play and Playfulness, *European Journal of Psychotherapy and Counselling*, 10(2): 121–129.

# 13

## PLAYFUL POLICY

*Rachel Bayliss and Alison Tonkin*

### Introduction

This chapter (which links to all other chapters in the book) will explore how play and playfulness, as an integral part of the policy agenda, can improve health and wellbeing through a shared mandate for public action. The Nuffield Council on Bioethics (2007: v) asks: 'Is it entirely up to us as individuals to choose how to lead our lives, or does the state also have a role to play?'

According to Barron and Cumberlege (2016), improving the health of the population is a major but necessary challenge for policy makers, although the potential rewards cannot be ignored. Public health is reliant upon politics, since governmental action is usually required for the delivery of outcomes (Oliver 2006). Coordinating the 'organized efforts of society' (Winslow 1920) requires a 'political community' with a shared bond between members which prompts collective action as opposed to individual endeavor (Oliver 2006). However, collective action can also create ethical tensions due to the constraints it places on 'individual choice' (Nuffield Council on Bioethics 2007).

In a political climate of accusation that the government acts as a 'nanny state' (Nuffield Council on Bioethics 2007), the self-reinforcing pleasure generated by play through the reward pathways of the brain (Perry et al. 2000) has been identified as an under-researched area of health, with much to contribute to the current public health agenda (Public Health Association of Australia 2018). Recognizing the negativity often associated with public health measures linked to 'moderating or even negating pleasure-seeking activities' (i.e. smoking, alcohol use, food choice and sexual activity), the Public Health Association of Australia (ibid.) advocates the promotion of pleasure as part of public health activity, stating that 'pleasure actually feels good, not only innately and individually, [but] also communally and collectively'.

## Background

The sentiment of a shared and universal opportunity of experience is central to effective public health policy. A principal tenet of Public Health England (2017a) has been to advocate the implementation of infrastructure that offers the 'same opportunities [to all] to lead a healthy lifestyle'. It has long been established that health is influenced by a kaleidoscope of interrelated factors which influence outcome, including: age, sex, socioeconomic status, environment, education and ethnicity. Healthcare inequalities are born out of differences in the experience of these variables and the inevitable social gradient which results (Marmot 2010). Policy acts as the building blocks from which fair opportunity can be sculpted. Essentially the focus is on 'levelling the playing field'; universal national policy objectives require tailoring for local delivery to meet the natural and socially constructed diversity of need and to close the inequality gap.

This cohesive equalizing strategy is echoed globally by the World Health Organization (WHO) who advocate 'an approach to public policies across sectors that systematically takes into account the health implications of decision, seeks synergies, and avoids harmful health impacts in order to improve population health and health equity' (WHO, cited in Public Health England 2016a). This characterizes the 'Health in All Policies' (HiAP) concept which demands a collaborative approach at a multi-tiered level (central, local, NHS, third party and private sectors), geared at incorporating health-related considerations into decision-making at policy level to address wider determinants of health (Public Health England 2016b).

It is evident that health and wellbeing concerns overlap many aspects of the policy agenda, as recognized by approaches such as the HiAP, and by a broader awareness of the influences of the wider determinants of health. It is therefore a natural step to appreciate the necessity and willingness for government budgeting and commissioning in this area, and the symbiotic relationship between funding and policy. With regards to play, government spending stems from an appreciation that policy is a necessary catalysing framework to facilitate united opportunities for leisure, recreation and sport, which can then serve as tools for promoting health and wellbeing in the context of the wider socio-political landscape. Karen Bradley, the Secretary of State for Culture, Media and Sport (CMS) in the UK, states that the benefits of activities under the remit of CMS 'has a value that goes beyond the economic':

> They matter in and of themselves. They raise the human condition and cheer our spirits – and the aggregate effect of individual experiences is to create a healthier, smarter, more peaceable, more cohesive and happier society.
> *(Karen Bradley, cited in Department for Culture, Media and Sport 2017: 9)*

Besides these anecdotal acclaims, there is also a body of academic research which resonates with policy aims in relation to health promotion, wellbeing and building resilience (HM Treasury 2003; Lester and Russell 2008). Funding allocation is influenced by such evidence, and supporting theory ultimately translates into provision and policy, albeit within a myriad of complicating, limiting factors and pressures. Although idealistic in nature, a helpful illustration of this relationship is the fluid triangle of analysis proposed by Lester and Russell (2008) as shown in Figure 13.1.

The triangular framework may be somewhat more nebulous in practice, but it creates a context for the rationale behind government spending and for the landscape in which plans to achieve health equality are sown.

## Leisure

The Committee on Culture, Science and Education (2005), meeting in 2005 as part of the Parliamentary Assembly for the Council of Europe, debated the report *Education for Leisure Activities*. Stating that the 'essence of politics' is to enhance the quality of life of the public and of the whole of society, the report provides strong advocacy for the role of governments, implying that the substantial benefits provided by leisure and recreational activities must be incorporated into the policy agenda. The report identified that the amount of time people spend working is gradually diminishing, in parallel with an increase in life expectancy and people having more free time at their disposal. The Committee on Culture, Science and Education (ibid.) stated that 'active participation in sport or music or other leisure activities can contribute to the improvement of health and to the strengthening of social cohesion' and 'governments are responsible for providing their citizens with conditions for the best possible quality of life…with leisure policy forming an indispensable element of State social policy', for all citizens irrespective of age, cultural or demographic differences.

With such an overwhelming endorsement of the integration of leisure and recreational activities and facilities into the policy framework of European governments, it is surprising that interventions and initiatives with play and playfulness at their heart are so often relegated in the political agenda (Knell and Taylor 2011), especially at a time when financial austerity invites the exploration of innovative solutions and interventions to pressing public health concerns. Despite a substantial evidence-base and a wealth of good practice examples, the role of playful endeavor is rarely identified in the context of enhancing public health.

Recognizing the creative arts as one of the diverse representations of play, reveals a rich evidence-base for the inclusion of playful endeavors linked to public

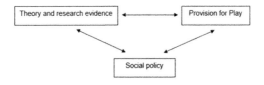

**FIGURE 13.1** Play, policy and practice: analytical framework.

health. In 2017, the All Party Parliamentary Group (APPG) on Arts, Health and Wellbeing published *Creative Health: The Arts for Health and Wellbeing*, following a two-year inquiry into the role of the Arts in health and social care in the UK. The aim was to provide recommendations that would improve policy and practice, through the collation of current examples of how the Arts are contributing to health and wellbeing through the life course (APPG on Arts, Health and Wellbeing 2017). The report noted that the importance of engagement with the Arts was often overlooked, and that there was an apparent 'blind spot' in recent health policy documentation, resulting in 'modest and limited' policy recommendations (ibid.). The APPG on Arts, Health and Wellbeing (ibid.) state they are not advocating legislative change or increased public spending, but support from Government to enable a process of change which acknowledges and promotes the creative arts as a means of enhancing the health and wellbeing of the population, both for the individual and for society (Lord Howarth of Newport, cited in APPG on Arts, Health and Wellbeing 2017). This reinforces Barron and Cumberlege's (2016:9) call for cross-government action, proposing 'a paradigm shift in policy, whereby health is seen as a fundamental component of a prosperous and sustainable society and a priority in all policy areas'.

## Integrating playful endeavors into public health policy

In 2008, the government's Foresight Mental Capital and Wellbeing Project (2008), which is discussed in detail in Chapter 2, commissioned the National Economics Foundation (NEF) to identify how mental capital could be improved. The subsequent report entitled *Five Ways to Well-being – Mental Capital* identified five evidence-based actions that promote wellbeing (Aked et al. 2008). These are summarized in Table 13.1 together with the potential benefits and associated play-based opportunities for promoting engagement.

According to the What Works in Wellbeing Center (cited in What Works Center for Wellbeing 2017) the Five Ways to Wellbeing already contribute to many of the activities we enjoy and care about. Since its introduction, Five Ways to Wellbeing has been used as an evaluation framework by local authorities when reviewing community wellbeing initiatives. In 2012, the European Social Survey (ESS) was the first major research project which included questions related to the five ways to wellbeing, enabling comparison in wellbeing behavior across Europe (What Works Center for Wellbeing 2017). Using the rich data collated by the ESS, Harrison et al. (2016: 7) identified that:

> Across the world, there is growing recognition that it makes sense to measure people's wellbeing and treat it as a central policy objective … [providing] a more democratic perspective on how we understand societal success, as it places people at the heart of the story.

The results showed that Scandinavian countries, which have the highest levels of wellbeing, also have the highest rates of participation in relation to the five ways of

**TABLE 13.1** The benefits from engaging with the five ways to wellbeing.

| Five simple steps | Benefits | Opportunities |
|---|---|---|
| Connect … | Developing relationships enriches life and brings support. | Engage with family, friends, peers, colleagues and neighbors. This can be through physical and creative activities that have a social element (i.e. Knit and Natter groups). |
| Be active … | Makes individuals feel good and maintain mobility. | Sports and active hobbies such as walking, gardening, cycling, playing games. |
| Take notice … | Noting everyday moments helps foster appreciation of what matters – particularly good for mental health. | Connection with the natural world, particularly green and blue space, walking to work or talking with friends. |
| Keep learning … | Gives satisfaction and boosts confidence – with the added benefit of being fun. | Learn to play an instrument or cooking favourite foods…set enjoyable challenges. |
| Give … | Helping others links individual happiness to the wider community and is very rewarding. | Participation in community life such as helping with Parkrun (see Chapter 12), the World's Biggest Coffee Morning, Comic Relief and other charitable fund-raising initiatives with a playful element. |

Source: adapted from Chief Cultural & Leisure Officers Association (2014); Aked et al. (2008)

wellbeing. Conversely those countries with the lowest rates of participation are shown to also have the lowest rates of wellbeing (Abdallah 2016).

Lovell and Bibby (2018) acknowledge that no single idea or policy will improve the health of the public on its own and that 'solutions require all members of society to acknowledge the health impact of what they do and work together to take action' (Lovell and Bibby 2018:45). Many of the play-based opportunities which contribute to well-being are based in the community, suggesting a key role for local authorities in their facilitation. The Chief Cultural & Leisure Officers Association (2014) emphasized that policy-makers should link cultural and leisure programmes to the public health agenda through the identification of how these programmes impact on five interrelated domains:

- *Health protection* – ensuring the population is protected from illness and injury.
- *Health Improvement* – offering services and environments that improve health and wellbeing.
- *Prevention of ill health* – reducing the number of people living with preventable diseases.
- *Healthy life expectancy* – preventing premature death and reducing differences in life expectancy between communities.
- *Wider determinants of health and inequalities* – the real domain where policy makers can create conditions that determine whether someone is healthy or not (ibid.).

The remainder of this chapter will explore how play and playfulness have been integrated into each domain, citing examples linked to policy initiatives at local, national and international levels.

## Health protection – health and safety

The Chartered Institute of Environmental Health (2017) defines health protection as 'the branch of public health concerned with policies and practice to improve the prevention and control of infectious diseases and other environmental threats to the health of the population'. The Chartered Institute of Environmental Health works collaboratively with the Health and Safety Executive (HSE) whose mission is to 'prevent death and ill health in Great Britain's workplaces' (HSE 2018a). Health and safety (H&S) is a vital tool for protecting health and wellbeing but is often treated with disdain and regarded as an irritant. Brown (2014) describes how health and safety often falls foul to 'terrible jokes and prejudice', citing 'the real reasons some people hate health and safety'. One of the reasons is that health and safety operatives are seen as a 'bunch of killjoys … intent on sucking joy out of the world' (ibid.). However, Brown goes on to explain that H&S operatives 'don't just tolerate fun activities – they actively encourage them … i.e. kayaking, mountain climbing and motor bike riding' (ibid.). Brown suggests that people need to be as 'safe as necessary, not as safe as possible', affirming that physical activity and enjoying life are essential for mental and physical wellbeing, and that sound H&S practice helps to facilitate this. Brown asks 'who's afraid of the big bad wolf?', noting that 'elf and safety' is an easy target for producing 'H&S bogeyman stories' (ibid.). Between April 2007 and December 2010, the HSE produced a *myth of the month*, which aimed 'to dispel some of the most widely believed health and safety myths' (HSE 2018b). Using humor and cartoon illustrations, the HSE debunked each myth, stressing that 'H&S' is an inaccurate and unhelpful reason for banning certain activities. Examples include:

- Children banned from playing conkers unless wearing safety goggles.
- Trapeze artists being forced to wear hard hats.
- Candy floss on a stick banned in case people trip and impale themselves on the stick.
- Graduates ordered not to throw their mortar boards in the air (HSE 2018c).

The HSE, while keen not to trivialize health and safety matters, identify these myths as 'ridiculous and baffling', stating that 'there is no shortage of daft decisions being blamed on health and safety' (HSE 2018c). By adopting a playful approach to dispel these false-truths, the HSE demonstrate an alternative way of raising awareness and generating discussion around H&S issues which enhances engagement in a novel and entertaining manner. The HSE continue to address H&S myths through the Myth Busters Challenge Panel who investigate cases where H&S has been incorrectly cited as a reason for an activity-ban, including categories linked to community and volunteering as well as sports and leisure.

## Health improvement – social prescribing

With current estimates suggesting a £30 billion funding gap between healthcare service need and delivery in the UK by 2020, the need to identify alternative public health innovations is high on the policy agenda. The drive for sustainability becomes even more significant in times of fiscal constraint and the concept of *social prescribing* is gaining recognition as a means of utilizing 'untapped potential for local and national action to support healthier lives' (Lovell and Bibby 2018).

Social prescribing enables the connection of 'people with local community services and activities [so] we can improve the health and wellbeing of large numbers of people', and local governments are ideally placed to facilitate this (Seccombe, cited in Local Government Association 2016). With a fifth of general practitioner (GP) visits now for social rather than medical reasons, GPs are being encouraged to 'refer patients with social, emotional or practical needs to a range of non-clinical services' such as those shown in Figure 13.2. Many of these activities have play and playfulness at their core.

Underpinned by the theoretical concept of salutogenesis (discussed in more detail in chapter 3), social prescribing identifies health as a positive state of wellbeing and recognizes factors that contribute to the creation of health and wellbeing as 'assets' (Health Education England 2016) that are frequently provided by community and charity-based organizations. These can include cooking, gardening, group-learning, healthy-eating activities, art activities, a range of sporting activities, as well as volunteering (King's Fund 2017). Philanthropy and charitable work also deliver a wide range of beneficial outcomes which enhance the health and wellbeing of those who volunteer or contribute financially, as well as of those who utilize the services, amenities and environments offered through the third sector.

Charities contribute to the operation and organization of society but have only a limited influence in terms of canvassing for policy change, particularly when evidence of efficacy is a prerequisite for inclusion in public policy. Bickerdike et al.

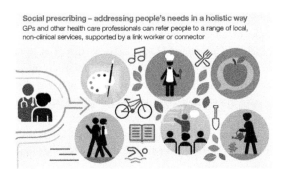

Social prescribing – addressing people's needs in a holistic way
GPs and other health care professionals can refer people to a range of local, non-clinical services, supported by a link worker or connector

**FIGURE 13.2** Social prescribing.
Source: Public Health England (2018a); Open Government Licence 3.0
(www.nationalarchives.gov.uk/doc/open-government-licence/version/3)

(2017) warn that, despite the obvious potential and wide support for social prescribing, there is currently insufficient evidence to evaluate the effectiveness of this
approach, in terms of success or value for money. As with so many play-based
approaches, it has proved difficult to define 'outcome measures' for the intangible
benefits and enjoyment provided by play, resulting in another 'blind spot' which
may limit subsequent policy recommendations in the future (APPG on Arts,
Health and Wellbeing 2017).

## Prevention of ill health – loneliness

As a social herd, humans are hard-wired to play; De Koven (2014: 160) notes that
'playfulness is one of the signs scientists look for when trying to determine the health
of a herd of animals. The healthier the animals and the safer the herd, the more they
play'. Lovell and Bibby (2018: 24) confirm that 'people who are more socially connected to family, friends and their community are happier and live longer, healthier
lives with fewer physical and mental health problems than people who are less well
connected' (discussed in detail in Chapters 5 and 7).

Loneliness is regarded as an evolutionary trait (Cacioppo et al. 2014) and
'separation from the herd' is experienced as an immediate threat to survival
(Breuning 2016). The perceived threat of harm through social isolation (loneliness)
is responsible for the release of the steroid hormone cortisol (ibid.), and sustained,
raised cortisol levels are associated with diseases such as cardiovascular disease, diabetes, cognitive decline and high blood pressure. These are all now identified as
corrosive health problems associated with chronic loneliness (Griffiths n.d.).

According to Griffin (2010: 4), loneliness 'is not being alone but a subjective
experience of isolation' – implying that loneliness is a perceived state of social isolation which is unique to the individual experiencing it. An admission of loneliness
carries social stigmatization, which serves to exacerbate and perpetuate the problem
(Khullar 2016). Historically, loneliness was regarded as a purely social or cultural
issue and efforts to mitigate it were limited by a lack of awareness of its potential
impact on health (Griffin 2010). Recent epidemiological evidence has been crucial
to raising awareness of the scale and consequences of loneliness, revealing its
influence on people of all ages, cultures, socioeconomic status and geographical
regions (Thomas 2018). Klinenberg (2018) suggests that it is not helpful to frame
increasing levels of loneliness as an 'epidemic', nor to focus on prevalence and impact
and that it has been the analysis of statistical data which has resulted in headline
stories, spurring people into action. This is exemplified by the appointment in 2018,
by the UK government, of a Minister for Loneliness (Mead 2018), reinforcing
Griffin's (2010: 7) assertion that 'one approach to loneliness is preventative: we can
stop loneliness becoming chronic and tackle the needs of groups that are socially
excluded and at risk of isolation'.

Initiatives designed to address social isolation can be very simple. *Be happy to chat*
encourages conversations with neighbors or with fellow shoppers in the super-
market queue, visits to elderly relatives or a friend who hasn't been seen for a long

time (Jo Cox Loneliness 2018). Play and playfulness can act as a catalyst for this social engagement, with activities such as those featured in Figure 13.1 presenting opportunities for people to meet one another on a regular basis to engage in shared interests and hobbies (Public Health England 2018a). This is further exemplified by the Men in Sheds project which offers a setting in which men can access support and develop friendships. This project is of potential benefit for single men as well as for those facing retirement, redundancy or widowhood – life changes which can often lead to social isolation (Lovell and Bibby 2018).

Play also has a role in nurturing and maintaining relationships, which in turn support and improve mental health (Reville 2015). Reville recommends having between three and five close friendships that involve face-to-face contact for optimal health, noting that non-kinship friendships are more beneficial to mental health than kin friendships with siblings or spouses (ibid.). However, Reville reminds that, despite its many health-related benefits, friendship should be 'pursued and cultivated for its own sake and not viewed as a form of social therapy' (ibid.).

## Healthy life expectancy and communities

Perhaps one of the most transparent indicators of public health is life expectancy. This ultimate measure depends on a multitude of factors, including the diversity of the community. *Community* itself is a fluid and evolving construct, a chameleon-like concept which can change dependent on the categories or boundaries applied to it (geographical, ethnic, cultural etc.). An added facet to the concept of life expectancy is *healthy life expectancy,* which adds a quality of life dimension to the length of the lifespan: the focus is shifted from pure existence to how well we live, a consideration directly influenced by play and leisure.

Since 2002, both life-expectancy and healthy life expectancy have increased and, according to Public Health England (2018a), the 'population is living longer and spending more years in good health'. In 2016, life expectancy in England reached 79.5 years for males and 83.1 years for females, of which self-assessed good health (2013–2015) was reported as 63.4 years for males and 64.1 years for females (Public Health England 2017b). In the context of an increasingly aging population, the Government Office for Science (2017) project Future of an Ageing Population provided 'state of the art' scientific evidence for the foundation of a range of policies that were intended to:

- 'maintain wellbeing throughout life, for all individuals regardless of their generation';
- 'improve quality of life for older people and enable them to participate more fully in society'; and
- 'ensure everyone can access the tools and facilities to help them live a long and healthy life' Government Office for Science (2017).

There is clear evidence that community has a vital role to play in achieving these intentions for people of all ages. Public Health England (2018a) advocates community as the very 'heart of public health', influencing 'health improvement, health protection and healthcare public health'. O'Mara-Eves et al. (2013) hail community engagement strategies as 'effective in improving health behaviors, health consequences, participant self-efficacy and perceived social support for disadvantaged groups'.

A working example of community engagement for health and wellbeing is the *Community development route to health improvement* in Aylesbury, England (UK Government 2018). This initiative revolves around a Healthy Living Center in the town center and promotes engagement in targeted areas of deprivation across the region. Specific activities nurtured by the scheme include: walking groups, a boxing club, the Silver Singers (a choir for those with dementia), a youth hub and educational programmes such as a 'skilled for health' maternity programme aimed at mothers from ethnic minorities. The project was born out of consultation and engagement work with the community to identify specific needs around promoting health and social support (UK Government 2018). The benefits are manifold in improving healthy life expectancy: the community is empowered, protective healthcare behaviors and educations cultured, loneliness reduced, and social participation and cohesiveness enhanced. People are connected to the community resources and activities around them with policy acting as a bridge between the potential availability of services and actual utilization. Community involvement sees the social and environmental barriers to leisure and play removed or lessened, opportunities widened, and vulnerable or minority groups brought under a sphere of influence they may not have previously enjoyed. In some respects, policy could be argued to 'open the eyes' of the community to the opportunities for play and leisure within it.

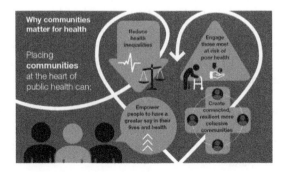

**FIGURE 13.3** The importance of communities for public health.
Source: Public Health England (2018a); Open Government Licence 3.0 (www.natio-nalarchives.gov.uk/doc/open-government-licence/version/3)

## Wider determinants of health and inequality

Accessibility and health inequalities share a complex inter-dependent relationship with the wider determinants of health. These determinants are a diverse line-up of environmental, socio-economic and personal factors which impact a person's health (Marmot 2010). It is here that policy once again steps into the frame as a powerful enabler 'governing local, national and international distribution of power and resources which shape the conditions of daily life' (Public Health England 2018b).

The universal nature of play and playfulness makes them potent weapons in the battle against inequality. The literature is peppered with examples of play and leisure provision making inroads into levelling the effects of the wider determinants of health. One such illustration is the Street Play Scheme. This has targeted 33 geographically diverse areas and involves temporary, controlled street closures to facilitate opportunities for urban outdoor leisure activities (Play England 2017). The scheme serves to reach areas of highest deprivation (often with less available green space) and seeks to maximize involvement by promoting social interaction and neighborliness. The Street Play vision is 'for every child to have the freedom to regularly play actively and independently in front of or near their own front door, contributing to a healthy lifestyle' (ibid.: 11). Evaluation has shown that the scheme results in greater physical activity – three times higher outdoors than in – with sedentary behaviors replaced by physical exertions (ibid.). Policy is central to the implementation of the Street Play Scheme, not only to navigate the bureaucratic complexity of organizing street closures, but to manage the convergence of safety, transport, planning and health issues in a controlled and appropriate manner. In this respect, it is *policy* that facilitates accessibility, allowing children and their families to engage with the environment in which they live for a greater health purpose.

The provision and spread of outdoor public gyms have similarly improved accessibility to opportunities for physical exercise with a wide range of secondary benefits. Lee et al. (2018) claim that outdoor gyms are increasingly recognized as an important strategy in 'realising the public health agenda of promoting physical activity'. By removing financial barriers to participation, and by relaxing time-restrictions (due to 24/7 availability), outdoor gyms represent the open-access potential of such initiatives with the added benefits for participants of exercising in the great outdoors. The public availability of outdoor gyms also removes barriers to participation for vulnerable or minority groups who may not previously have had access to such services.

Outdoor gyms have also spawned innovative means of training in the use of the exercise facilities, including scannable QR codes used to deliver equipment instructions on smartphones and free weekly inductions run by qualified gym instructors for members of the public (Brent Council 2018). Ease of access, the possibility of incorporating exercise into the daily routine, and encouragement through cross-generational utilization create a convincing mandate for more outdoor gyms (Sharing.Lab 2017). The funding, maintenance and promotion of these outdoor gym facilities necessitates bolstering by policy, not only in terms of budgeting and set-up, but for continued investment in upkeep and awareness-raising (ibid.).

Leisure policy which addresses disparities in the wider determinants of health is also evident in the cultural realm of museums. In December 2001, British government policy dictated free access to all the permanent collections of the national museums. In recent years, 'the use of arts and culture to deliver other policy goals' has identified museums as a positive contributor 'to a range of social priorities, including health, education, community engagement, and social inclusion' (Mendoza 2017). This notion chimes with the Happy Museum project (Happy Museum 2018) which credits museum visitation with increased general happiness and self-reported health. Following the policy change on entry fees, the MORI survey identified that, in addition to a generalized increase in museum visits, there was a modest rise from 20–25 per cent in visitors from more deprived social classes, opening-up a previously more restrictive cultural domain (MORI 2003).

Certain museums have additionally cultivated local projects to build upon government policy and promote social cohesion and healthcare improvements. The Manchester Museum launched a project designed to embed playfulness into its wider appeal by incorporating play opportunities for visitors and promoting playful encounters within the museum space (Happy Museum 2016). Targeting the opposite end of the age spectrum, the National Museum in Liverpool created a 'House of Memories', with object-based therapy and educational workshops for people with dementia and their carers (see http://houseofmemories.co.uk).

These are just two examples of nationwide initiatives which recognize the health and wellbeing benefits of cultural inclusion and which reflect the underlying government policy of wider engagement.

## Conclusion

This chapter has journeyed through the actual and potential application of play and leisure as a fundamental component of the policy agenda. Embedded in public health policy is the established human right that everyone has a right to leisure and play. Playful policy becomes the key that opens the door of opportunity to shared and cohesive leisure experiences which address healthcare inequalities by catering for variations in the wider determinants of health. The cited examples of current policy initiatives demonstrate a focus on harnessing community empowerment and utilizing the natural environment to achieve healthcare goals. These resonate with the jigsaw of international recognition that nothing less than a holistic approach to public health is required.

Policy is a necessary manifestation of the government's responsibility to facilitate a maximum achievable healthy life expectancy and quality of life for the whole population. This is with the caveat that the spontaneity inherent in play should not be undermined by unnecessarily excessive regulation. Achieving an effective balance between policy and practice is a precarious and dynamic process, open to complex pressures and influences, a path best navigated with an open and receptive attitude to new evidence and evolving theory. As Gilmore (2016: 17) suggests: 'We need to give our legislators the courage and support to act to improve the nation's health without spoiling all the fun.'

# References

Abdallah, S. (2016) Fives Ways to Wellbeing, in E. Harrison, A. Quick and S. Abdallah (eds), *Looking through the Wellbeing Kaleidoscope*, 41–50, London: New Economics Foundation.

Aked, J., Marks, N., Cordon, C. and Thompson, S. (2008) *Five Ways to Wellbeing*, London: New Economics Foundation.

APPG on Arts, Health and Wellbeing (2017) *Creative Health: The Arts for Health and Wellbeing* [The Short Report], London: All Party Parliamentary Group on Arts, Health and Wellbeing.

Barron, K. and Cumberlege, J. (2016) *A Healthier Life for All: The Case for Cross-Government Action*, London: The Health Foundation.

Bickerdike, L., Booth, A., Wilson, P., Farley, K. and Wright, K. (2017) Social Prescribing: Less Rhetoric and More Reality. A Systematic Review of the Evidence, *BMJ Open*, 7: e013384, retrieved from https://mafiadoc.com/social-prescribing-bmj-open_59dda c331723ddae41636ba1.html (accessed 20 May 2018).

Brent Council (2018) Outdoor Gyms, retrieved from www.brent.gov.uk/outdoorgyms (accessed 30 April 2018).

Breuning, L. (2016) Do You Want to Share Your Pain or Relieve It?, retrieved from www. slideshare.net/LorettaBreuning/do-you-want-to-share-your-pain-or-relieve-it (accessed 6 April 2018).

Brown, L. (2014) The REAL Reasons Some People HATE Health and Safety, retrieved from https://rospaworkplacesafety.com/2014/06/19/hate-health-and-safety (accessed 14 April 2018).

Cacioppo, J.Cacioppo, S. and Boomsma, D. (2014) Evolutionary Mechanisms for Lone-liness, *Cognition & Emotion*, 28(1), retrieved from Http://doi.org/10.1080/02699931. 2013.837379 (accessed 7 June 2018).

Chartered Institute of Environmental Health (2017) Health Protection, retrieved from www.cieh.org/policy/health_protection.html (accessed 14 April 2018).

Chief Cultural & Leisure Officers Association (2014) The Role of Culture and Leisure in Improving Health and Wellbeing, National Leisure & Culture Forum.

Committee on Culture, Science and Education (2005) Report: Education for Leisure Activities, retrieved from www.assembly.coe.int/nw/xml/XRef/X2H-Xref-ViewHTML.asp?FileID= 10971&lang=EN (accessed 9 April 2018).

De Koven, B. (2014) *A Playful Path*, ETC Press.

Department for Culture, Media and Sport (2017) *Annual Report and Accounts: For the Year Ended 31 March 2017*, London: Department for Culture, Media and Sport.

Foresight Mental Capital and Wellbeing Project (2008) *Systems Maps: Mental Capital and Wellbeing Project*, London: Government Office for Science.

Gilmore, I. (2016) Harm from Alcohol: The Solutions Are There But Not the Will to Implement Them, in *A Healthier Life for All: The Case for Cross-Government Action*, 16–17, London: The All-Party Parliamentary Health Group and the Health Foundation.

Government Office for Science (2017) Collection: Future of Ageing, retrieved from www. gov.uk/government/collections/future-of-ageing#project-report (accessed 21 May 2018).

Griffin, J. (2010) *The Lonely Society?*, Mental Health Foundation.

Griffiths, H. (n.d.) *Social Isolation and Loneliness in the UK: With a Focus on the Use of Technology to Tackle These Conditions*, IoTUK.

Happy Museum (2016) Case Study – Real Practice, Real Impact Manchester Museum – Developing Skills to Support Child-Led Play, retrieved from http://happymuseump roject.org/wp-content/uploads/2010/02/HM_case_study_Manchester_WEB_Mar2016. pdf (accessed 30 April 2018).

Happy Museum (2018) Principles, retrieved from http://happymuseumproject.org/about/why/principles (accessed 7 June 2018).

Harrison, E., Quick, A., and Abdallah, S. (eds) (2016) *Looking through the Wellbeing Kaleidoscope*, London: New Economics Foundation.

Health Education England (2016) *Social Prescribing at a Glance North West England: A Scoping Report of Activity for the North West*, Health Education England.

HM Treasury (2003) Policy Paper: Every Child Matters, retrieved from www.gov.uk/government/publications/every-child-matters (accessed 30 April 2018).

HSE (2018a) Inside HSE, retrieved from www.hse.gov.uk/aboutus/insidehse.htm (accessed 14 April 2018).

HSE (2018b) Myth of the Month, retrieved from www.hse.gov.uk/myth/mythofthemonth.htm (accessed 14 April 2018).

HSE (2018c) Top 10 Worst Health and Safety Myths, retrieved from www.hse.gov.uk/myth/top10myths.htm (accessed 14 April 2018).

Jo Cox Loneliness (2018) Young or Old, Loneliness Does Not Discriminate, retrieved from www.jocoxloneliness.org/pdf/a_call_to_action.pdf (accessed 21 May 2018).

Khullar, D. (2016) How Social Isolation Is Killing Us, *The New York Times*, 22 December, retrieved from www.nytimes.com/2016/12/22/upshot/how-social-isolation-is-killing-us.html (accessed 25 January 2018).

King's Fund (2017) What is Social Prescribing?, retrieved from www.kingsfund.org.uk/publications/social-prescribing (accessed 20 May 2018).

Klinenberg, E. (2018) Is Loneliness a Health Epidemic?, *The New York Times*, 9 February, retrieved from www.nytimes.com/2018/02/09/opinion/sunday/loneliness-health.html (accessed 4 April 2018).

Knell, J. and Taylor, M. (2011) *Arts Funding, Austerity and the Big Society: Remaking the Case for the Arts?*, London: RSA.

Lee, J., Lo, T. and Ho, R. (2018) Understanding Outdoor Gyms in Public Open Spaces: A Systematic Review and Integrative Synthesis of Qualitative and Quantitative Evidence, *International Journal of Environmental Research*, 15: 590.

Lester, S. and Russell, R. (2008) *Play for Change*, London: Play England.

Local Government Association (2016) *Just What the Doctor Ordered Social Prescribing – a Guide for Local Authorities*, London: Local Government Association.

Lovell, N. and Bibby, J. (2018) *What Makes Us Healthy? An Introduction to the Social Determinants of Health*, London: The Health Foundation.

Marmot, M. (2010) Marmot Review Executive Summary: Fair Society, Healthy Lives, retrieved from www.instituteofhealthequity.org/resources-reports/fair-society-healthy-lives-the-marmot-review/fair-society-healthy-lives-exec-summary-pdf.pdf (accessed 29 April 2018).

Mead, R. (2018) What Britain's 'Minister of Loneliness' Says About Brexit and the Legacy of Jo Cox, *The New Yorker*, 26 January, retrieved from www.newyorker.com/culture/cultural-comment/britain-minister-of-loneliness-brexit-jo-cox (accessed 21 May 2018).

Mendoza, N. (2017) *The Mendoza Review: An Independent Review of Museums in England*, Department for Digital, Culture, Media & Sport.

MORI (2003) Impact of Free Entry to Museums, retrieved from www.culturehive.co.uk/wp-content/uploads/2013/04/Impact-of-free-entry-to-museums-MORI.pdf (accessed 30 April 2018).

Nuffield Council on Bioethics (2007) *Public Health: Ethical Issues*, London: Nuffield Council on Bioethics.

Oliver, T. (2006) The Politics of Public Health Policy, *Annual Review of Public Health*, 27(1): 195–233.

O'Mara-Eves, A., Brunton, G., McDaid, D., Oliver, S., Kavanagh, J., Jamal, F.Matosevic, T., Harden, A. and Thomas, J. (2013) Community Engagement to Tackle Inequalities, retrieved from www.ncbi.nlm.nih.gov/pubmed/25642563 (accessed 7 September 2018).

Perry, B., Hogan, L. and Marlin, S. (2000) Curiosity, Pleasure and Play: A Neurodevelopmental Perspective, *HAAEYE Advocate*, August: 9–12.

Play England (2017) *Why Temporary Street Closures for Play Make Sense for Public Health*, London: Play England.

Public Health Association of Australia (2018) Pleasure and Health – A Colloquium, 15 June 2018, retrieved from www.phaa.net.au/about-us//pleasure-and-health-a-colloquium-15-june-2018 (accessed 15 March 2018).

Public Health England (2016a) Health in all Policies Slideset, retrieved from www.gov.uk/government/publications/local-wellbeing-local-growth-adopting-health-in-all-policies (accessed 7 May 2018).

Public Health England (2016b) Health in All Policies: Local Wellbeing, Local Growth, retrieved from https://assets.publishing.service.gov.uk/government/uploads/system/uploads/attachment_data/file/560598/Health_in_All_Policies_overview_paper.pdf (accessed 30 April 2018).

Public Health England (2017a) Understanding Health Inequalities in England, retrieved from https://publichealthmatters.blog.gov.uk/2017/07/13/understanding-health-inequalities-in-england/ (accessed 29 April 2018).

Public Health England (2017b) Research and Analysis: Chapter 1: Life Expectancy and Healthy Life Expectancy, retrieved from www.gov.uk/government/publications/health-profile-for-england/chapter-1-life-expectancy-and-healthy-life-expectancy (accessed 21 May 2018).

Public Health England (2018a) Wider Determinants of Health Interactive Tool, retrieved from https://fingertips.phe.org.uk/profile/wider-determinants (accessed 30 April 2018).

Public Health England (2018b) Health Matters: Community-Centred Approaches for Health and Wellbeing, retrieved from www.gov.uk/government/publications/health-matters-health-and-wellbeing-community-centred-approaches/health-matters-community-centred-approaches-for-health-and-wellbeing (accessed 30 April 2018).

Reville, W. (2015) Loneliness: The Next Big Global Health Problem? *The Irish Times*, 16 April, retrieved from www.irishtimes.com/news/science/loneliness-the-next-big-global-health-problem-1.2169996 (accessed 6 April 2018).

Sharing.Lab (2017) The Rise of Outdoor Gyms: Nudging People to Be More Active, retrieved from https://medium.com/we-research-and-expriment-with-how-the-sharing/the-rise-of-outdoor-gyms-nudging-people-to-be-more-active-a1b3babe97f8 (accessed 22 May 2018).

Thomas, J. (2018) Loneliness is a Growing Social Problem. We Must Tackle This Major Public Health Concern, retrieved from www.thenational.ae/opinion/comment/loneliness-is-a-growing-social-problem-we-must-tackle-this-major-public-health-concern-1.697209 (accessed 6 April 2018).

UK Government (2018) Case Study: Community Development Route to Health Improvement in Aylesbury, retrieved from www.gov.uk/government/case-studies/community-development-route-to-health-improvement-in-aylesbury (accessed 30 April 2018).

What Works Centre for Wellbeing (2017) Five Ways to Wellbeing in the UK, 18 January, retrieved from https://whatworkswellbeing.org/blog/five-ways-to-wellbeing-in-the-uk (accessed 14 April 2018).

Winslow, C. (1920) The Untilled Fields of Public Health, *Science*, 51(1306): 23–33.

# 14

## PLAYFUL ENDINGS

### Making meaning at the end of life

*Julia Whitaker and Alison Tonkin*

### Introduction

Play and playfulness are fundamental to the human condition, and the concept of a playful ending 'highlights the humanity that lies within all of us, at any stage of life ...' (Ellis and Zeedyk 2014). Dame Cicely Saunders, founder of the modern hospice movement, affirms this with eloquent simplicity in the statement, 'You matter because you are you, and you matter all the days of your life' (Cicely Saunders International 2013).

This chapter explores how the authenticity found in the freedom of creative play can inform our perspectives on death and dying, and how the merging of play and playfulness with end-of-life experiences offers an alternative approach to understanding and supporting those at the end of life's journey. A public health approach to the end of life demands more than just a services approach because it also necessitates a reorientation of our attitudes and behaviors towards death, dying, loss, and palliative care, and hinges on community participation (Karapliagou and Kellehear 2013). Hannah (2014: 106) observes that, 'modern society does not have a vibrant myth about death, which can make it more difficult for us to face'. Finding a place for playfulness on the public health agenda, adds to the repertoire of available options at the end of life and creates the potential for a different way of death.

### Play as authenticity

If there are points in our lives when we can be said to be truly ourselves, they are at the very start and at the very end of life. The newborn is transparent in their motives, feelings and actions (Zeedyk and Robertson 2011) and this transparency re-emerges at life's end when there is no longer a need or a desire to consciously act a part, to conform, or to satisfy the expectations of others. At the end of life, as at its start, there is a synergy between all parts of the person and 'we are truly liberated to be the persons we are meant to be' (Chan 2006: 56). In 'The Ontology of Play', Fink (1960: 101) writes that play is 'just as original and basic in itself as death …' in the sense that both play and death allow for the emergence of the truly authentic self. In play, as at life's ending, we enter a zone of authenticity in which we are free to be completely ourselves, a state imbued with 'exciting and precarious' possibilities (Winnicott 1971).

The concept of 'authenticity', and its relationship to wellbeing, has been the subject of scholarly interest for centuries and has been conceptualized in various ways, but it is a concept heavily influenced by humanism and self-determination theory (Mengers 2014). Maslow (1968) famously cites authenticity as a higher-order psychological need, essential for the ultimate experience of self-actualization by which we transcend the opinions of others to become truly ourselves. Authenticity balances the human drive for belonging with the need to be perceived as unique (Vignoles 2009) – both traits regarded as fundamental to the achievement of wellbeing. Mengers (2014: 53) proposes that 'the development of more open and accepting societies can encourage people to be more authentic and unique, potentially creating well-being on both an individual and community level.' Thus, the extent to which we are free to have an 'authentic' end to our lives is inextricably linked to the social and cultural context of our dying.

Historically, the rituals surrounding death and dying were central to community life and identity: end of life practices were guided by cultural traditions and the performance of rituals which 'brought together a cast of actors in the performance of clinical, psychological, spiritual and social care' (Karapliagou and Kellehear 2013). Heidegger (1994) locates true playfulness in this communal enactment of the myths, rituals and practices which represent belonging to a unique time, place, and social group. Seasonal festivities, religious ceremonies and public celebrations serve to transport the participant away from the busy certainty of the everyday, to a place of mystery and wonder in which the fragility of life is experienced with unquestioning acceptance. Grondin (2001:44) explains: 'when we are playfully concerned with something, we are also seriously there with "sacred seriousness"'. Active participation in the 'sacred seriousness' of play frees us to experience the true essence of life and of ourselves in the world (Gadamer 1984).

Active participation in play and playfulness also contributes to the development of the social capital essential for the creation of healthy communities when it reinforces existing relationships based on trust, empathy and community cooperation. The ritual celebrations associated with entering and leaving the world have traditionally been authentically playful and at the start of the 21st century there emerges a new-found playfulness in social attitudes to death and dying and thus a new potential for building 'healthy settings' (World Health Organization 1986) linked to 'ecological environments, habitats and people' (Karapliagou and Kellehear 2013).

## Re-engaging societal participation at the end of life

The World Health Organization (2017) 'regards dying as a normal process': it is the one thing of which we can all be certain. Karapliagou and Kellehear (2016: 154) have conservatively estimated that each year, in England alone, around 2 million people will be directly engaged in activities associated with 'dying, caregiving and bereavement' – yet death and dying remain 'significant social taboos ... that [are] frequently perceived as "too difficult" for individuals, communities and civic society to discuss and so dying is not given priority' (National Council for Palliative Care n.d.). However, the idea of death as the 'ultimate taboo' is a relatively modern concept (Gorer 1965).

At the start of the 20th century, most people died at home and communities accepted the reality of death, and care of the dying, as everyday aspects of community life (Karapliagou and Kellehear 2013). A gradual shift to hospital-based dying over the past hundred years has seen death and dying removed from common experience: during this period, hospital deaths peaked at 90 per cent of the total in some parts of the West (Collins 2017). The move away from reliance on the socially supportive participation of the local community at the end of life has been accompanied by a reluctance to acknowledge the importance of 'dying well' – both for the person who is dying and for those who care for them. This undermines the fact that 'how people die remains in the memory of those who live on' (Saunders cited in Potts 2016). Research indicates that many people find the process of caring for someone at the end of their life to be an isolating and stressful experience, to the detriment of their own physical and mental wellbeing (Collins 2017). Kinderman (2017) advocates the collective creation of a more humane society which minimizes psychological health problems and promotes wellbeing for all. Compassion is a fundamental human response which enables us to share the suffering of others through the demonstration of 'social empathy, acceptance and understanding' (Karapliagou and Kellehear 2013: 37) and the creation of compassionate communities depends on a partnership model which stresses our interconnectedness.

The challenge to public health posed by an aging population and the ever-increasing prevalence of dementia-related conditions in the elderly population, has presented opportunities to revisit public attitudes to care at the end of life and to ensure that compassion is at the core of health and care practices. The Netherlands is renowned for its innovative models of social care (Brindle 2017), and the growing practice of multi-generational residential care is one model which has garnered international attention (International Observatory on Social Housing n.d.). At the residential and care center Humanitas in Deventer, university students live alongside the elderly residents, participating in the musical arts committee, assisting staff therapists, and volunteering at seasonal events in exchange for free accommodation. Their day-to-day interactions with their elderly housemates are imbued with play and playfulness as they share 'the little joys of everyday life' (Jansen 2015) – watching films and sport, playing music and games, and sharing stories of their respective lives (YouTube 2016). The Humanitas center also pioneers the practice of 'dementia whispering' as a way of maintaining close emotional connection at the close of life (YouTube 2018). This style of non-verbal communication uses physical closeness and touch to facilitate the authentic expression of playfulness and joy at what is more typically a time of disconnection and sorrow (Ellis and Zeedyk 2014).

Compassionate, connected communities are communities which preserve a place for play right-up to the end of life.

Collins (2017) advocates innovation, as demonstrated by multigenerational care in the Netherlands, to achieve better outcomes at the end of life for all concerned. Seymour (2017) asserts that the arts and humanities 'have a role to play in allowing individuals and communities to express experiences of illness, death, and grief and encourage conversation and thoughtful reflection'. Recognition of the innovative potential of play and playfulness in this context represents a dynamic contribution to this public health debate. Many of the core activities of public health, such as health promotion, public education and community engagement remain relevant to end of life experiences and may serve to facilitate a return to the active community participation demanded of a compassionate community. Compassionate communities minimize social isolation, offer support to carers (Collins 2017), and provide services which recognize the value of life to its end-point, including the contribution that the dying 'may still want to make to [their] families, work or community' (National Council for Palliative Care n.d.).

This has become more achievable in recent years with the advent of social media as a vehicle for sharing personal stories that open-up conversations about sensitive subjects. Rachel Bland, a BBC radio presenter, was diagnosed with breast cancer in 2016 and documented her 'cancer journey' through her blog *Big C Little Me* and through the podcast *You, Me and the Big C: Putting the Can in Cancer,* with Lauren Mahon and Deborah James (Davies 2018). At the time of her death in September 2018, the podcast had reached number one in the iTunes podcast listings (iTunes Charts 2018) and much of this success was attributed to 'the show's bold humor … the presenters know that it helps draw people into a subject that might otherwise be too difficult to contemplate' (Rogers 2018). Messages of support for Bland's family on Twitter after her death exemplify how fun and humor were crucial in opening-up frank conversations which have been an inspiration to so many (BBC Radio 5 Live 2018).

Public health is traditionally associated with society's efforts to protect the health of the public, promoting better health for all and preventing ill health. A public health approach to death and dying aims to improve the health and wellbeing of individuals at the end of life, through encouraging communities to develop their own approaches to death, dying, loss and caregiving (Karapliagou and Kellehear 2013). However, 'interest in the social experience and epidemiology of end of life experiences is extremely low' (Karapliagou and Kellehear 2016: 153) in comparison to other public health activities such as smoking cessation or reducing obesity.

## Playing with death

De Koven (2014: 164) declares: 'Dying isn't fun. Being dead, in all likelihood, is not fun. Someone else's death, even a pet's death, is not fun. And yet, and yet playing dead is immensely fun.'

Death themes have pervaded children's play throughout history and across cultures (Opie and Opie 1969), from the infant's peek-a-boo (from the old English meaning 'alive or dead') to depictions of violent destruction in contemporary video games. Children's natural curiosity and their use of play as a means of exploration and discovery (Perry et al. 2000) mean that from an early age they can conceptualize death as part of life, and how life and death fit together (Dying Matters n.d. a). In his seminal research into children's perceptions of death, Rochlin (1967: 54) notably concluded that 'death is a matter of deep consideration to the very young child' and children seem to have no difficulty finding the playfulness in death, whether that of themselves or of others.

Julia offers the following example from her caseload as a child and family therapist: a six-year-old child who was nearing death from respiratory disease. A regular feature of their twice-weekly hospital 'play visits' was a game in which the child would hide under the bedcovers while their visitor pretended to search for them:

> When the suppressed giggles could no longer be ignored, I would ask, 'Just what are you doing under there …?' and [they] would always answer, 'I'm *burying* myself with my blanket, of course!' It seemed to me that this repeated exchange was one way in which this child was trying to make sense of what was happening to [them].

Another case example is that of a child with a life-limiting cerebral tumour who played a never-ending game in which a 'child' puppet chased a 'robber' puppet across a series of insurmountable obstacles, the 'robber' always managing to evade capture. Julia reflects: 'I never worked-out whether this child identified with the pursuer or with the one trying to get away, but in a way that was irrelevant – this game was clearly a way of playing out the sad reality that death was fast catching-up with this child.'

The readiness of children to play around with the concept of death does not endure into adulthood, by which time the topic of death becomes a conversation-stopper. According to the National Council for Palliative Care (2016), only one in ten people have talked to somebody else about how or where they would like to die. Planning for one's own death seems to go against the survival instinct. To quote writer and filmmaker Woody Allen, 'It's not that I'm afraid to die, I just don't want to be there when it happens' (Allen 1975: 99).

The Dying Matters Coalition (Dying Matters 2018) is an example of how partnership with 'community groups, organizations and coalitions [can] support strategies that promote public health' by developing and implementing educational campaigns to extend knowledge, understanding and the exploration of attitudes (PublicHealthCareerEDU.org 2017). The Dying Well Community Charter, published by the National Council for Palliative Care (n.d.) promotes collaborative approaches to death and dying, stating that 'care for one another at times of crisis and loss, is not simply a task for health and social care services but is everybody's responsibility'. The Charter highlights the importance of open, honest communication as an indicator of respect, compassion and understanding. Openness shares features with play in that its outcome is unpredictable, which may explain why talking openly about death and dying is perceived as a risky business.

One of the many causes of social isolation is the fear of saying the wrong thing and of eliciting a negative or distressing emotional reaction. Silk and Goldman (2013) have formulated a technique for 'how not to say the wrong thing', based on the Ring Theory of 'kvetching' (Jimma 2016). *'Kvetching'* is a Yiddish term meaning to continuously moan, grumble, groan or complain (ibid.). This approach is designed to protect the 'aggrieved or afflicted' and those closest to them from well-meaning others who may unintentionally allow free expression to their own needs and feelings, rather than offering selfless and unconditional support (ibid.). The 'ring theory', illustrated in Figure 14.1, proposes that, while anyone may offer comfort and support to the 'sad or sick' person portrayed at the center of a series of concentric circles of influence, people may only kvetch (or 'dump') on those further removed from the target person than themselves. Silk and Goldman (2013) identify this as an extension of our natural inclination to avoid burdening those under stress with our own concerns, despite the temptation to offer personal opinion or advice. 'People who are suffering trauma don't need advice. They need comfort and support' (ibid.) and play and playfulness represent an alternative, uniquely supportive, means of maintaining connection and communication when words are hard to find. Listening to music, singing, sharing a story,

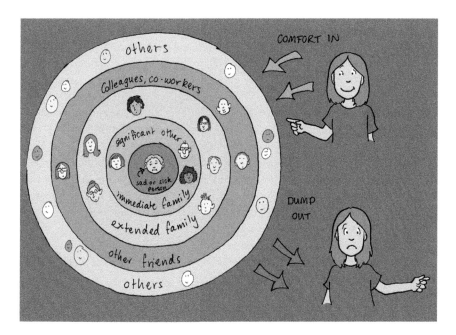

**FIGURE 14.1** Ring theory of kvetching.
Source: Lizzy Mikietyn (adapted from an illustration by Wes Bausmith, cited in Silk and Goldman 2013)

looking through family photographs, playing a card game or doing a puzzle together all demonstrate selfless care and compassion. Play allows everyone to be present in the moment – even at the very final moment.

## The funeral as play

Play and ritual may both be described as 'meta-action' (Stromberg 2009) in that they are concerned with ideas and symbols and meta-level commentary on everyday happenings (Heller cited in Magister 2017). Play is a way of framing, or reframing, and interpreting everyday life in order to reveal what is important or authentic about the experience. Both play and ritual transcend the physical reality of death and loss and, in so doing, they represent complementary frames (Handelman 2013) for making meaning of death. The funeral is both ritual and play with its own cast of characters, script, properties and setting, and is imbued with a social and cultural power for collective meaning-making. The nature of the funeral ritual varies across history and culture and many funerary practices are recognizably playful, incorporating music, dancing and feasting (Torgovnick May 2013).

- The New Orleans Jazz Funeral is perhaps one of the most widely recognized for its joyful, boisterous expression of grief (Funeralwise 2018).
- The Mexican *Dia de Muertos* (Day of the Dead) is celebrated as a public holiday: 'a three-day fiesta … filled with marigolds, the flowers of the dead; *muertos* (the bread of the dead); sugar skulls; cardboard skeletons; tissue paper decorations; fruit and nuts; incense, and other traditional foods and decorations' (Day 2003: 72).
- The African tradition of *nine nights*, still practised in the Caribbean, includes the playing of dominos and other games, and concludes with a dramatic rendition of a traditional folk tale (Williams 2015).
- A sense of optimistic humor is evident in the Korean tradition of *kkoktu*: funerary figures designed to be 'fun and friendly – even kind of cute' companions on the journey to the afterlife (Schwendener 2007). These anthropomorphic figures typically include the character of the 'entertainer' whose role is to console the deceased and to distract mourners from their grief. In the words of Schwendener: 'We're all joining that party eventually, and it might be nice to have a few clowns and acrobats, even a monk on a turtle leading the way' (ibid.).
- In his book *Island of Bali*, Covarrubias (2015: 325) writes in a similar vein that, 'strange as it seems, it is in their cremation ceremonies that the Balinese have their greatest fun.'

The concept of the 'fun funeral' (I Want a Fun Funeral 2017) has found resonance with a generation of millennials, who are noted to be more 'open-minded than their parents on controversial topics' (YouGov 2013) and whose approach to social change is characterized by a 'pragmatic idealism', unrelated to religious affiliation (Burstein 2013: 3).

Attitudes to death, like other cultural mores, have been subject to the impact of cultural globalization. Across the world, people are challenging traditional approaches to death, and experimenting with creative alternatives to long-established beliefs and practices. From 'build-your-own-coffin' clubs in New Zealand (Somvichian-Klausen 2017) to death cafés (e.g. http://deathcafe.com) serving up conversation and cake in over 50 countries, there appears to be a new willingness to 'play around' with what has been regarded as one of life's most sacred rituals of transition (Funeral Source 2017). There has been a noticeable cultural shift from the sombre church ceremony towards more playful 'celebrations of life' which might include popular music, bubbles, balloons or fireworks. In a 2011 survey commissioned by Co-operative Funeral Care, 54 per cent of respondents said they would opt for a celebration of life, rather than a simple church service, and 48 per cent would want their funeral to reflect their favourite hobby, color, football team or music (Co-operative Press 2017). Bespoke coffins, including a Lancaster bomber, Doctor Who's Tardis, and a yacht, are nothing if not playful and echo the figurative palanquins and fantasy coffins which have been a feature of Ghanaian culture since the early 20th century (Tschumi 2014).

## The playful memorial

There are similarly playful changes to the ways in which societies choose to remember the dead. The Future Cemetery project represents an acknowledgement that 'the disposal of human remains extends beyond the purely corporeal to increasingly digital and virtual remnants of a human life' (see http://futurecem etery.org). From a design-winning skyscraper cemetery in Norway (Orange 2013), and egg-shaped memorial tree urns from Italy (Capsula Mundi 2016), to LED Buddhas in Japan (Jozuka 2016), a spirit of playfulness is evidenced in these creative and challenging alternatives to the ways in which the dead have traditionally been memorialized.

The expansive application of digital media has also played a part in transforming the ways in which people remember the dead and choose to communicate about end of life matters. In 2009, the National Council for Palliative Care set up the Dying Matters Coalition (Dying Matters 2018) to promote public awareness of issues around dying, death and bereavement. Dying Matters (n.d. b), TalkDeath (2016a) and the 'death positive' movement are examples of a growing number of digital forums which encourage greater openness around the subject of death through the sharing of information and personal stories and signposting to other resources. Digital technology has also increased the range of commemorative alternatives, including memorial profiles on social media, livestreams and memorial DVDs (Bruce 2015). There is an argument to be made that, in an era dominated by electronic media, many people may find the anonymity of virtual communication a preferable option when exploring difficult topics (Whitaker and Weldon 2016).

Art has always offered 'a different way of seeing and talking about things we'd rather not discuss' (Rankin cited in Dying Matters 2016) and in 2016, Dying Matters launched a photography competition, Celebrate Life in the Face of Death, as an alternative way of approaching 'the reality of death for all of us, and then to celebrate the life we have' (Dying Matters 2016). This reflects a centuries-old artistic preoccupation with death (TalkDeath 2016a) from depictions of funeral procession scenes in Plague Art and the *danse macabre* of the 16th century, to the expressionism of Van Gogh's *Wheatfield with Crows* and the literal representations of the postmodernists, including Warhol and Hirst (Silka 2017). The concept of authenticity in art rests on an understanding that it represents a true expression of the values and beliefs of the individual or of society (Dutton 2003) and play and art overlap in this capacity for synthesizing the essence of what is meaningful at any particular time and place. Grondin, in his analysis of Gadamer's discourse on art as play, writes: 'The play of art does not lie in the artwork that stands in front of us, but lies in the fact that one is touched by a proposition, an address, an experience, which so captures us that we can only play along.' (Grondin 2001: 43).

In 2017, BBC Radio 4 broadcast a feature about musician and sculptor Nick Reynolds (BBC 2017), who has revived the centuries-old tradition of creating death masks. The art of the death mask has been described as 'a stepping stone between an animate being and the inert corpse … an interface rather than a face' (Funeral Alternatives 2017). Reynolds found a focal point for his own grieving when he created a death mask of his father, enabling him to talk to his father while accepting the fact of his physical death. He has subsequently revived and developed the craft, sculpting death-like images of both the famous and the infamous. This exposes how the artistic representation of the dead can give form to the abstract concept of death, facilitating both grieving and remembrance: 'the representation of death makes it understandable, graspable and tangible' (Øygarden Flæten and Rasmussen 2015: 126).

The death motif also pervades the music genre and is present in musical forms as diverse as church and classical music, folk songs, the Blues, and the so-called *coffin songs* of the 1950s and early 1960s (Pacholski 1986). In 2016, the Canadian Rock band, *The Tragically Hip*, broke new ground with their *Man Machine Poem* tour which marked the impending death of lead singer, Gord Downie, and demonstrated 'the communal power of music to break down the social disposition of fearing death *just* enough to acknowledge it' (TalkDeath 2016b). The power of popular music to engage groups of people in conversations about death is further illustrated by the 2016 publication of an open 'thank-you letter' which palliative care consultant, Dr Mark Taubert, wrote to rock legend David Bowie (Taubert 2016). In the letter, he detailed how the late star's music had inspired a conversation with a cancer patient facing the end of her own life. The widespread sharing of Taubert's letter on social media sparked a worldwide debate about how we approach end-of-life conversations, demonstrating both a need and a readiness to discuss this universal stage of development. Taubert opined that, 'celebrity death seemed to be an acceptable way "in" to the big conversation about how people want to face the last months and years of their lives' (Taubert 2017), a phenomenon spectacularly displayed following the death of Diana, Princess of Wales, in 1997, when collective mourning was enacted on a global scale.

## Conclusion

As humans, we live our whole lives in the knowledge that one day we shall die: no other animal has the same capacity for looking towards the future (Kets de Vries 2016). Yet this knowledge is accompanied – at least in the West – by a tendency to deny it or, at least, to keep it at a distance. In a youth-obsessed society, which places the greatest value on the wealth-generating potential of the young (James 2007), death becomes something to avoid at all costs. Modern healthcare systems regard death as a failure, as an affront to their designated purpose (Hannah 2014). The denial of death as a psychologically and socially significant part of life serves to compromise opportunities for reflection and re-evaluation with associated risks for the whole of society (Kets de Vries 2016). A preparedness to challenge the status quo and to acknowledge the possibilities for a more *playful ending* to life represents a fresh and more hopeful approach to the ways in which society addresses this life-stage with greater authenticity:

> Like anything else we need to understand, especially when it comes to big, hurting things that are too big, too painful to grasp, death and dying are things we need to play with. Over and over again. Not because we need to understand them. But because it's the only way we can even begin to accept them as real.
>
> *(De Koven 2014: 164)*

## References

Allen, W. (1975) *Without Feathers*, New York: Random House.

BBC (2017) Death Masks: The Undying Face, retrieved from www.bbc.co.uk/programm es/b0939wgs (accessed 30 November 2017).

BBC Radio 5 Live (2018) Mother to Freddie … Twitter, 5 September, retrieved from https:// twitter.com/bbc5live/status/1037279327858118656 (accessed 6 September 2018).

Brindle, D. (2017) Buurtzorg: the Dutch Model of Neighbourhood Care that Is Going Global, *The Guardian*, 9 May, retrieved from www.theguardian.com/social-care-network/ 2017/may/09/buurtzorg-dutch-model-neighbourhood-care (accessed 5 September 2018).

Bruce, R. (2015) The Best Way to Utilize Technology for Memorials, retrieved from www. thedigitalbeyond.com/2015/12/the-best-way-to-utilize-technology-for-memorials (accessed 3 December 2017).

Burstein, D. (2013) *Fast Future: How the Millennial Generation is Shaping Our World*, Boston, MA: Beacon Press.

Capsula Mundi (2016) Life Never Stops, retrieved from www.capsulamundi.it/en (accessed 8 September 2018).

Chan, S. (2006) *Liturgical Theology: The Church as Worshiping Community*, Intervarsity Press.

Cicely Saunders International (2013) Putting Patients and Families First: Making Sense of the Independent Inquiry into the Liverpool Care Pathway, retrieved from www.kcl.ac. uk/nursing/departments/cicelysaunders/attachments/lcp-press-release–cicely-saunder s-international-150713.pdf (accessed 8 December 2017).

Collins, J. (2017) Dying Well is a Public Health Issue, The Ravens Daily Blog, 12 October, retrieved from www.publicsectorexecutive.com/The-ravens-daily-blog/dying-well-is-a -public-health-issue (accessed 8 December 2017).

Co-operative Press (2017) The Changing Face of 'Co-op' Funerals, retrieved from www.the news.coop/36085/sector/retail/changing-face-co-op-funerals (accessed 21 November 2017).

Covarrubias, M. (2015) Island of Bali, North Clarendon, VT: Tuttle Publishing.

Davies, G. (2018) Rachael Bland, BBC Presenter and Cancer Blogger, Dies Two Days after Bidding 'Au Revoir' to Friends, The Telegraph, 5 September, retrieved from www.tele graph.co.uk/news/2018/09/05/rachael-bland-bbc-presenter-cancer-blogger-dies-two-da ys-bidding (accessed 6 September 2018).

Day, F. (2003) Latina and Latino Voices in Literature, Westport, CT: Greenwood Publishing Group.

De Koven, B. (2014) A Playful Path, ETC Press.

Dutton, D. (2003) Authenticity in Art, in J. Levinson (ed.), The Oxford Handbook of Aesthetics, 258–274, New York: Oxford University Press.

Dying Matters (2016) New Competition Challenges People to Photograph 'the Toughest Subject', retrieved from www.dyingmatters.org/news/new-competition-challenges-peop le-photograph-toughest-subject (accessed 6 September 2018).

Dying Matters (2018) About Us, retrieved from www.dyingmatters.org/overview/about-us (accessed 6 September 2018).

Dying Matters (n.d. a) What Should You Tell Children about Death, retrieved from www. dyingmatters.org/sites/default/files/user/images/Resources/Promo%20materials/Leaflet_ 8_Web.pdf (accessed 6 September 2018).

Dying Matters (n.d. b) Life is for Living, retrieved from www.dyingmatters.org/sites/defa ult/files/user/images/Resources/Promo%20materials/Leaflet_1_Web.pdf (accessed 6 September 2018).

Ellis, M. and Zeedyk, S. (2014) Rethinking Communication: The Connected Baby Guide to Advanced Dementia, Dundee: Suzanne Zeedyk.

Fink, E. (1960) The Ontology of Play, Philosophy Today, 4(2): 95–109.

Funeral Alternatives (2017) Death Masks & Who Commissions Them, retrieved from www.funera lalternatives.co.uk/2017/09/14/death-masks-commissions (accessed 30 November 2017).

Funeral Source (2017) The History of Funerals, retrieved from http://thefuneralsource.org/ history.html (accessed 21 November 2017).

Funeralwise (2018) New Orleans Jazz Funeral Service Rituals, retrieved from www.funera lwise.com/customs/neworleans (accessed 5 September 2018).

Gadamer, H.-G. (1984) Truth and Method, New York: Crossroad.

Gorer, G. (1965) Death, Grief, and Mourning in Contemporary Britain, New York: Doubleday.

Grondin, J. (2001) Play, Festival and Ritual in Gadamer: On the Theme of the Immemorial in his Later Works, in L. Schmidt (ed.), Language and Linguisticality in Gadamer's Hermeneutics, 43–50, Lanham, MD: Lexington Books.

Handelman, D. (2013) Play and Ritual: Complementary Frames of Meta-Communication, in A. J. Chapman and H. C. Foot (eds), It's a Funny Thing, Humour: Proceedings of The International Conference on Humour and Laughter 1976, 185–192, Amsterdam: Elsevier.

Hannah, M. (2014) Humanising Healthcare: Patterns of Hope for a System under Strain, Fife: International Futures Forum.

Heidegger, M. (1994) Basic Questions of Philosophy: Selected Problems of Logic, trans. R. Rojcewicz and A. Schuwer, Bloomington, IN: Indiana University Press.

International Observatory on Social Housing (n.d.) How the Dutch Lead the Way in Senior Housing Innovation, retrieved from https://internationalsocialhousing.org/2017/05/29/lea rning-best-practices-in-housing-for-the-elderly-from-the-dutch (accessed 5 September 2018).

iTunes Charts (2018) UK Podcasts: Current Top 10, retrieved from www.itunescharts.net/ uk/charts/podcasts (accessed 6 September 2018).

I Want a Fun Funeral (2017) Let's Talk, retrieved from www.iwantafunfuneral.com/lets-talk (accessed 12 March 2018).

James, O. (2007) *Affluenza*, London: Vermillion.

Jansen, T. (2015) The Nursing Home That's Also a Dorm, retrieved from www.citylab. com/equity/2015/10/the-nursing-home-thats-also-a-dorm/408424 (accessed 5 September 2015).

Jimma (2016) The Ring Theory of 'Kvetching' or 'How Not To Say The Wrong Thing', retrieved from http://beyondgoodbye.co.uk/?p=6419 (accessed 13 December 2017).

Jozuka, E. (2016) Death Is a High-Tech Trip in Japan's Futuristic Cemeteries, retrieved from https://motherboard.vice.com/en_us/article/9a3a5a/death-is-a-high-tech-trip-in-japa ns-futuristic-cemeteries (accessed 23 November 2017).

Karapliagou, A. and Kellehear, A. (2013) *Public Health Approaches to End-of-Life Care: A Toolkit*, London: Middlesex University.

Karapliagou, A. and Kellehear, A. (2016) The Forgotten People in British Public Health: A National Neglect of the Dying, Bereaved and Caregivers, *BMJ Supportive & Palliative Care*, 6: 153–159.

Kets de Vries, M. (2016) *Sex, Money, Happiness and Death*, New York: Palgrave Macmillan.

Kinderman, P. (2017) Creating a More Humane Society, in All Party Parliamentary Group for Health, *A Healthier Life for All: The Case for Cross-Government Action*, 26–27, London: The Health Foundation.

Magister, C. (2017) The Connection between Ritual, Art and Play. Burning Man Project, retrieved from https://journal.burningman.org/2017/03/philosophical-center/the-them e/the-connection-between-ritual-art-and-play (accessed 21 November 2017).

Maslow, A. (1968) *Toward a Psychology of Being*, 2nd edition, New York: D. Van Nostrand.

Mengers, A. (2014) The Benefits of Being Yourself: An Examination of Authenticity, Uniqueness, and Well-being, retrieved from https://repository.upenn.edu/cgi/view content.cgi?article=1064&context=mapp_capstone (accessed 24 November 2017).

National Council for Palliative Care (2016) *Dying Matters Coalition: Public Opinion on Death and Dying*, London: Comres.

National Council for Palliative Care (n.d.) The Dying Well Community Charter: Principles of Care and Support, retrieved from www.ncpc.org.uk/sites/default/files/Dying_Well_ Community_Charter.pdf (accessed 6 September 2018).

Opie, P. and Opie, I. (1969) *Children's Games in Street and Playground*, Oxford: Oxford University Press.

Orange, R. (2013) 'Vertical Cemetery' Wins Praise for Originality, retrieved from www. thelocal.no/20131128/vertical-cemetery-commended-at-oslo-grave-conference (accessed 23 November 2017).

Øygarden Flæten, J. and Rasmussen, T. (2015) *Preparing for Death: Remembering the Dead*, Göttingen: Vandenhoeck and Ruprecht.

Pacholski, R. (1986) Death Themes in Music: Resources and Research Opportunities for Death Educators, *Death Studies*: 10(3): 239–263.

Perry, B., Hogan, l. and Marlin, S. (2000) Curiosity, Pleasure and Play: A Neurodevelopmental Perspective, *HAAEYE Advocate*, August: 9–12.

Potts, J. (2016) In Praise of the Hospice: 'How People Die Remains in the Memory of Those Who Live On', *The Telegraph*, 22 August, retrieved from www.telegraph.co.uk/ health-fitness/body/in-praise-of-the-hospice-how-people-die-remains-in-the-memory-of (accessed 8 December 2017).

PublicHealthCareerEDU.org (2017) Public Health Education and Health Promotion, retrieved from www.publichealthcareeredu.org/public-health-education (accessed 13 December 2017).

Rochlin, G. (1967) *How Younger Children View Death in Themselves*, in E. A. Grollman (ed.), *Explaining Death to Children*, 51–73, Boston, MA: Beacon Press.

Rogers, J. (2018) You, Me and the Big C: 'When you Talk about Cancer, You Normalise It', *The Guardian*, 10 June, retrieved from www.theguardian.com/tv-and-radio/2018/jun/10/you-me-and-the-big-c-interview-rachael-bland-lauren-mahon-deborah-james (accessed 8 September 2018).

Schwendener (2007) Korea's Extraordinary Send-Offs for Ordinary People, retrieved from www.nytimes.com/2007/08/17/arts/design/17kore.html (accessed 12 March 2018).

Seymour, J. (2017) The Impact of Public Health Awareness Campaigns on the Awareness and Quality of Palliative Care, *Journal of Palliative Medicine*, 1(20) (Suppl. 1): S30–S36.

Silk, S. and Goldman, B. (2013) How Not to Say the Wrong Thing, *Los Angeles Times*, 7 April, retrieved from http://articles.latimes.com/2013/apr/07/opinion/la-oe-0407-silk-ring-theory-20130407 (accessed 8 September 2018).

Silka, P. (2017) How Art Dealt with Death Throughout its History, retrieved from www.widewalls.ch/death-art (accessed 28 November 2017).

Somvichian-Clausen, A. (2017) Kiwi Coffin Club Throws Glitter on the Idea of Dying, from https://news.nationalgeographic.com/2017/10/new-zealand-coffin-club-death-music-spd (accessed 21 November 2017).

Stromberg, P. (2009) *Caught in Play: How Entertainment Works on You*, Stanford, CA: Stanford University Press.

TalkDeath (2016a) The Six Most Popular Depictions of Death in Art, retrieved from www.talkdeath.com/the-six-most-creative-depictions-of-death-in-art (accessed 28 November 2017).

TalkDeath (2016b) Dead Man Walking: Canadians Face Death with The Tragically Hip, retrieved from www.talkdeath.com/dead-man-walking-canadians-face-death-with-the-tragically-hip (accessed 28 November 2017).

Taubert, M. (2016) A Thank You Letter to David Bowie from a Palliative Care Doctor, retrieved from http://blogs.bmj.com/spcare/2016/01/15/a-thank-you-letter-to-david-bowie-from-a-palliative-care-doctor (accessed 29 November 2017).

Taubert, M. (2017) Bowie and the Lazarus Effect, *Remedy*, 24, retrieved from www.cardiff.ac.uk/__data/assets/pdf_file/0007/538693/remedy_edition_24.pdf (accessed 29 November 2017).

Torgovnick May, K. (2013) Death Is Not the End: Fascinating Funeral Traditions from Around the Globe, retrieved from https://ideas.ted.com/11-fascinating-funeral-traditions-from-around-the-globe (accessed 21 November 2017).

Tschumi, R. (2014), *Concealed Art. The Figurative Palanquins and Coffins of Ghana*, Bern: Edition Till Schaap.

Vignoles, V. (2009) The Motive for Distinctiveness: A Universal, but Flexible Human Need, in S. J. Lopez and C. R. Snyder (eds), *The Oxford Handbook of Positive Psychology*, 491–500, Oxford: Oxford University Press.

Whitaker, J. and Weldon, C. (2016) Using Play as a Means to Widen Access to Health and Well-being, in A. Tonkin, and J. Whitaker (eds), *Play in Healthcare for Adults: Using Play to Promote Health and Wellbeing Across the Adult Lifespan*, 70–84, Abingdon: Routledge.

Williams, P. (2015) The Death of Nine Nights – Part 1, retrieved from http://jamaica-gleaner.com/article/news/20150531/death-nine-nights-part-1 (accessed 21 November 2017).

Winnicott, D. (1971) *Playing and Reality*, London: Routledge.

World Health Organization (1986) *The Ottawa Charter for Health Promotion*, Geneva: World Health Organization.

World Health Organization (2017) WHO Definition of Palliative Care, retrieved from www.who.int/cancer/palliative/definition/en (accessed 8 December 2017).

YouGov (2013) The Sun Survey Results, retrieved from http://cdn.yougov.com/cumulus_uploads/document/jgdvn3vm4b/YG-Archive-Pol-Sun-results-190613-youth-survey.pdf (accessed 2 December 2017).

YouTube (2016) Drinking Games and Jigsaws: A Unique Dutch Retirement Home, retrieved from www.youtube.com/watch?v=_KWwso1CQPw (accessed 5 September 2018).

YouTube (2018) Dementia Whispering: A New Way to Treat Degenerative Disease?, retrieved from www.youtube.com/watch?v=92E_2nJkSjw (accessed 5 September 2018).

Zeedyk, S. and Robertson, J. (2011) *The Connected Baby*, DVD, Dundee: Connected Baby.

# INDEX